IF

THE BUDDHA

CAME

TO DINNER

IF
THE BUDDHA
CAME
TO DINNER

HOW TO NOURISH
YOUR BODY TO AWAKEN
YOUR SPIRIT

Halé Sofia Schatz
with SHIRA SHAIMAN

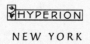

NEW YORK

Library of Congress Cataloging-in-Publication Data

Schatz, Halé Sofia.
    If the Buddha came to dinner: how to nourish your body to awaken your spirit / Halé Sofia Schatz, with Shira Shaiman.
        p. cm.
    Includes bibliographical references.
    ISBN 0-7868-6883-X
    1. Nutrition. 2. Spirituality. I. Shaiman, Shira. II. Title.
RA784 .S382   2003
613.2—dc21   2002032707

Hyperion books are available for special promotions and premiums. For details contact Michael Rentas, Manager, Inventory and Premium Sales, Hyperion, 77 West 66th Street, 11th floor, New York, New York 10023, or call 212-456-0133.

FIRST EDITION

10 9 8 7 6 5 4 3 2 1

Nurture the spirit
Be sparing with energy
As though holding a full bowl

Sun Bu-er, twelfth-century Taoist master

To my children, Micah, Josef, and Yasemin,
who are loved from a deep well of nourishment.
May your lives be an inspiration for others.
And for Steven, who keeps my heart.

May all spirits be deeply nourished.

CONTENTS

ACKNOWLEDGMENTS *XI*

INTRODUCTION *1*

PART ONE: WHO ARE YOU FEEDING?

1. TRANSFORMATIONAL NOURISHMENT *15*

2. THE WAKE-UP CALL *31*

3. EMBODYING SPIRIT *49*

PART TWO: NOURISHMENT AS DAILY PRACTICE

4. VITAL ESSENCE FOODS *65*

5. DAILY PRACTICE *83*

6. THE CLEANSE: A RETREAT INTO YOURSELF *111*

PART THREE: AWAKENING YOUR SPIRIT

7. DISCIPLINE: THE ROOT OF FREEDOM *153*

8. LIVING YOUR RHYTHM *163*

9. BECOMING A SOURCE OF NOURISHMENT *175*

PART FOUR: RECIPES FROM THE HEARTH

INTRODUCTION TO RECIPES *191*

GLOSSARY OF INGREDIENTS *297*

SELECTED BIBLIOGRAPHY *301*

ACKNOWLEDGMENTS

Numerous people have supported and inspired the creation of this book. Without my family's unconditional support, this work would not have come into being. With deep gratitude and love, I wish to acknowledge my husband, Steven, who has been my partner and advocate in actualizing the heart of nourishment for nearly thirty years. For the innumerable ways he joyously gave his attention and guidance and graciously kept our lives going while this project came into being, I thank him and thank him again. For being a continual source of nourishment for me, I thank my children, Micah, Josef, and Yasemin, Ellie and Norman Schatz, Aunt Rosie, Valihe and Orhan Bayçu, my *nene* Salihe, Aunt Lamia, and Uncle Vecdi.

Many friends and colleagues have generously provided guidance and inspiration, among them Deepbluewindhorsewoman, Deepblackjaguarwoman, and Deepbrownmudwoman, Myla and Jon Kabat-Zinn, David Ludwig, Lama Surya Das, Cheryl Richardson, Michael Gerrish, André Gregory, and Cindy Kleine.

I am profoundly appreciative of the brilliant mind and loving soul of my collaborator, Shira Shaiman. In Shira I found a trusted friend and colleague with the uncanny ability to understand, synthesize, and organize my life's work into a form that can reach far beyond the limits of my office. I can't imagine a more harmonious collaboration, or one filled with more laughter, lightheartedness, delicious meals, or shared joy of Krishna Das, whose inspired chanting we listened to for countless hours and must certainly infuse every page of this book. Without Shira's incredible ability to translate this ancient material into modern language, this book would still be a good idea hiding somewhere in my heart. This relationship is a blessing from God. And for that, I am deeply grateful.

I learned quickly that writing recipes is no small task, and I am enormously appreciative of Aimee Shifman's inspired contributions to Recipes from the Hearth. Aimee invested hundreds of hours and brought her passion for cooking and fantastic organizational skills together to help create these exquisite recipes.

Many hours went into client interviews and transcriptions, and for their abiding good help I am appreciative of Sara Kopf Levine, Ying Yu, and Yasemin Schatz.

To my trainees, the Women of Wisdom, who journeyed with me this year and committed themselves to this work, including testing recipes, Ginger Burr, Brenda Fingold, Pamela Gregory, Sara Kopf Levine, Caroline Lindeke, Liz Linder, Lynne Meterparel, Leslie Miller, Roberta Orlandino, Merriann Panarella, Patricia Prior, Aimee Shifman, and Ying Yu. I am most grateful to all the other recipe testers, George Mandler, Susan Mead, Amy Hannes, Ilana Fleisher, Jeannie Smith, and Josef Schatz.

For their visual assistance with the cover, I am grateful to Kate Canfield and Micah Schatz. For their artistic contributions, I am thankful to Liz Linder Photography and to Lisa Sawlit.

A sincere thank you to Jean Chalmers, Monica Dimino, Ellen Grosman, Ismail Çakaloz, Ayça Çerman, Yasuko Nakai, Fumiko Matsuura, Michi Kondo, Larry Shaiman, Jackie Fearer, Ray and Barbara Bane at Star Lookout House, Holly Bishop, Tom McNeely, Jessica Chang, Michael Noyes, and Ginza Restaurant and Kei Okada for their assistance throughout many stages of this project.

ACKNOWLEDGMENTS

To all my clients, thank you for trusting me to be part of your courageous journey along the path of nourishment, and for sharing your stories here.

I offer my heartfelt gratitude to my literary agent, Colleen Mohyde of the Doe Coover Agency, who believed in this project from the very beginning. I want to thank Bob Miller at Hyperion for his generous support and for having a visceral response to this nourishment work. Finally, I am grateful to my editor, Mary Ellen O'Neill, for giving me a great deal of freedom to write, providing invaluable editorial direction at just the right time, and for trusting the work to try it in her own home.

IF
THE BUDDHA
CAME
TO DINNER

INTRODUCTION

It's April in New England. I've been spending time in my garden, clearing away the dead leaves, pruning, getting ready to plant. Where I live in the suburbs of Boston, I have room only for a modest garden. Yet even in this relatively small space life abounds. When you turn the iron handle and walk through the large, white gate, you enter a meadow of wildflowers and peach and apricot trees. Continue following the path around the side of the house, and you'll find the garden with its mulberry tree, roses, plums, raspberry bushes, grape arbor, kiwis, and little rows of spring and summer vegetables. But all of that is to come later. Today, it's still early spring, and as I survey my garden I decide it's time to prune the grapevine.

This morning I pick up the clippers and set to work, just as I've done for many years. You have to *prune* a plant in order for it to *grow*. I find pruning to be very satisfying; I love the sure, swift sound of the clippers rhythmically slicing through a branch. With each cut, I know I'm clearing away the dead matter to make room for new growth. Periodic pruning isn't just for plants; it's a natural rhythm for all of us. Cleaning your closets, organizing your personal papers, getting rid of clutter, and spring-cleaning are all forms of pruning. I find that when the weather is warmer, people naturally recommit to living more active and healthy lives, which starts with internally pruning the parts of their lives that no longer nourish them. This internal pruning helps you discover your hidden potential for growth.

The grapevine looks lifeless in April, like dry, twisted sticks. I snip away at the branches on the sides of the arbor, and then reach up to clip the coiling tendrils above my head. And then the most amazing thing occurs. The vine begins to drip. From each cut, a drop of liquid beads up and then falls as another and yet another glistening drop forms. Of course, I'm not surprised; I knew to expect this. But in the early morning sunlight, the sight of those brilliant drops cascading from the vine is glorious.

The grapevine reminded me that we should never underestimate the power of life force. Until I cut the branches, there was no way to know that so much life was coursing through what appeared to be a dead plant. As soon as the vine was cut, you could see tangible proof of life in the pearly drops that rained down from the branches. And in only a few weeks, leaves will bud and open, beginning the growth cycle for a whole new season. If you garden, then you're familiar with this potent life force; you know how it will generate magnificent fruit if you just give the plant some attention and support.

This same life force exists within each of us. You might call it soul, God, Christ, or Buddha nature. I will use "spirit" to describe this sacred life-giving force, since this word can apply most universally without connoting any one spiritual practice. No matter the language we use, this energy is real and vital. It's our essential makeup. Our spirit is abundant in its gifts. In fact, its sole purpose is to help us make connections, heal, and be our truest selves. Our spirit is the place within ourselves that is balanced, connected to the source of life, where we are at home. Deep within us exists a well of nourishment where we can find the sustenance to live joyful and meaningful lives. All that's asked of us is *to know* that it exists, and then *to feed* this place within ourselves.

We eat every day, all day long. But we are eating on the run, grabbing a doughnut and a cup of coffee on our way to work, heating up TV dinners, or making meals from instant foods. According to *Fast Food Nation,* Eric Schlosser's thorough investigation of our country's fast-food preoccupation, about 90 percent of the money Americans spend on food goes toward purchasing processed food. In the incredible pace of our lives and with the availability of every prepackaged food imaginable, we have lost the connection between what we eat, why we feed ourselves, and how we feel. For the most part, people eat without a great deal of thought beyond the taste. But the simple, daily act of eating has the potential to become a profound catalyst for spiritual growth, from experiencing a renewed sense of vitality and purpose in life to discovering our true vocations and making deeper connections in all of our relationships.

This book is about going to the heart of your true self where the source of nourishment is always available to you. How do we regularly nourish our spirit so that it continually bears fruit? How do we literally feed this part of ourselves? Imagine for a moment that the Buddha is coming to dinner. What would you prepare? Most likely you wouldn't run out for fast-food burgers and onion rings. Instead, you'd spend time shopping and preparing the freshest, most tasty, wholesome meal you could produce with your very own hands, in your very own kitchen.

Now let's imagine that you are a spiritual being—which you are!—what would you feed yourself?

When I ask people this question, it usually catches them off guard, except for the die-hard chocolate lovers who would feed the entire world only chocolate if given their choice. Aside from them, people typically shrug and say they just don't know. The usual response goes something like this: "I guess I wouldn't eat what I normally do, but I'm not sure what I would eat instead." Sandwiches, bagels, pasta, potato chips, fried foods, coffee, and soda just don't seem like cuisine for the divine. What would you feed yourself if you were a spiritual being isn't supposed to be a trick question, but answering it requires you to be in touch with your spirit and to know how to respond to its needs. Only then can you nourish your body, heart, mind, and spirit with the care and awareness you deserve.

If the Buddha Came to Dinner is a guide to learning how to feed your spirit so that you can be fed by it on a regular basis. Nourishment isn't a one-way street; rather, think of it as a loop. Let's take a look at how the nourishment cycle works by returning to the garden for a moment. It would be unrealistic for me to think that my garden could yield all of the vegetables and fruits it does without my efforts. It's fairly straightforward. A garden can only grow if there's a gardener to prune, fertilize, seed, and regularly care for the soil and plants.

It's actually not very different for people. If we want our spirits to soar and direct our lives in rich and meaningful ways, we need to feed ourselves with the nourishing foods, activities, and relationships that encourage growth. What would happen if you treated your whole self—body, heart, mind, and spirit—as a garden worthy of your love and diligent efforts? What dead matter would you clear away? What would you plant? How would you fertilize the soil and nurture the seedlings? What will you do with this plentiful harvest from your garden?

WHAT IS NOURISHMENT?

When we are nourished, we know who we are. We know how we feel. We understand our priorities. We have a clearer understanding of our deep purpose in life. We have the freedom to act in a way that honors our truest self. When we are nourished, we move through life with graceful strength rather than helplessly reacting to the winds and storms that may blow our way. If you can listen *and* respond to the inner messages of your spirit, then you're in a state of nourishment. On the one hand, nourishment is food, yet food alone will never be enough to nourish us. Supermarket shelves are overflowing, but in this country we are starving for more. We are hungry for the nourishing foods and activities that feed our bodies, hearts, minds, and spirits as one integrated being.

From the time I was a young girl, I have been aware of nourishment as a daily practice. I spent the first eight years of my life in Istanbul. My memories of Turkey all have to do with the smells, sounds, sights, and tastes of food. From the time I was a toddler I practically lived in the kitchen, where my mother, grandmother, and aunts could keep an eye on me. From my seat, I would watch the elaborate and ancient dance of women preparing food to feed their family, which was directed by my grandmother, my *nene*, who most definitely was in charge of the kitchen.

Every morning we would go to the outdoor market to buy the fresh produce, fish, and meat for that day. The day's meals depended on what the earth had yielded. We bought bread from the local ovens, piping hot. When I was old enough, it was my job to get the bread. I loved this daily chore, walking home with the fresh loaf under my arm, warming my whole body. I always broke off the crusty end and ate it during the five-minute walk home. Under the tutelage of my grandmother, mother, and favorite aunt, I learned how to use all my senses to select the freshest vegetables and fruit in the market. I came to understand that the best, ripest produce carries a certain vibration— in its color and texture you can feel that it had been picked within hours. When I bit into the peach that we bought from the nearby orchard, the flavor and nectar burst in my mouth. I could taste the sun, rain, and earth in that piece of fruit. I could feel its life force.

Those happy hours in the kitchen were my first encounter with the hearth of nourishment. I loved the regular rhythms of marketing, cooking, and leisurely eating our meals together every evening with our cousins and other relatives who always dropped by. These rhythms connected me to my family and to my community. I intuitively understood that food's nourishing capacity far exceeded basic physical survival. Food had the power to bring a family together, to connect me to the earth and our planet's cycles, to nurture all my senses.

TRANSFORMATIONAL NOURISHMENT

When we begin to properly nourish our bodies, an amazing transformation takes place: We begin to discover ways for nourishing all parts of ourselves. This is *transformational nourishment*, the process of transforming habitual, constricting patterns and behaviors into nourishing practices that encourage growth and development. Is it really possible that *food* can help us live fuller, more aware lives? The answer is yes! Healthy foods alone won't enlighten you. In fact, they, too, can become an obsession. The key to transformational nourishment is awareness.

Transformational nourishment isn't a quick-fix food program; it's a set of tools for living an aware life. There are myriad paths for learning self-awareness, from religious traditions and faiths to yoga, meditation, and other spiritual disciplines. In general, however, the connection between food and spiritual development has not been widely explored. Most food models available today tend to focus only on the physical or emotional levels, such as dieting and eating disorders. Transformational nourishment's unique approach turns food and eating into a daily practice for becoming physically, emotionally, and spiritually aware.

The natural human inclination is to continually grow, change, and create. Even as you read this sentence, great biochemical changes are occurring within your body. Millions of cells are being created and dying, and we aren't close to being aware of it. Growth is a constant for all levels of life, from the cellular to the cosmic. So, too, as humans, our natural state is one of growth and change. But sometimes we get stuck. In our culture, we particularly run into problems because we are living more sedentary lives, and we eat the sweet, sticky, salty, highly refined foodstuffs that perpetuate a sedentary existence. These foods also tend to trap us in places where we feel safe, secure, and resistant to change.

When we are clear about our intention of how we want to develop, the foods that propel us forward usually are the ones that we don't crave. I've been a nourishment consultant for over twenty-five years and I've never seen a client who has addictive patterns with vegetables or lean proteins, such as tofu, fish, and organic meat. It may seem simple, but just by shifting your food consumption to more vital essence foods (vegetables, fruit, grains, lean proteins), you will feel more empowered and in touch with a deeper part of yourself.

While transformational nourishment is a subtle, nonlinear process, it's helpful to break it down into its multiple parts so you can see how the physical, emotional, and spiritual interconnect. As you start to eat clean food, the body responds by eliminating what isn't necessary. Depending on the individual, many types of physical changes can manifest over time—from greater energy and clarity of mind to improved digestion, weight loss, disappearance of allergies, and a strengthened immune system. At the same time, a similar process has been triggered on the emotional and spiritual levels. Negative emotional and behavioral patterns may also reveal themselves as "toxic." Maybe your self-perceptions, relationships, or how you've been living your life no longer support the person you are today, or the person you genuinely wish to become. When the body and emotions are unbalanced, we can't hear the voice that is our spirit, the deeper consciousness that we know to be true. With the body and emotions in a balanced, receptive state, the spiritual part of ourselves is more accessible.

To make lasting changes, you need both awareness and action. Just as something is dying, something new is being born. To make room for your new self, you have to prune the old patterns. Letting go is risky business because the old patterns, the old shell, seem so secure. The choice is yours. You can exert a lot of energy trying to resist your growth, or you can respond to the messages from your spirit.

Deidre first came to see me because she was in a medical crisis. She weighed 250 pounds and could hardly walk. She was on the brink of needing surgery in both of her knees, and was running out of options when a colleague recommended she see me. We worked together for seven months, and during that time she lost seventy pounds and her knees were almost pain-free without surgery. In our sessions, we explored who she used to be when her body didn't carry all the extra weight. She remembered that she used to feel potent, creative, and passionate, but these feelings had been muted for a very long time.

As Deidre shed the layers of weight that she had been carrying for many years, she began to get in touch with that creative and passionate part of herself again. She came to the painful though welcome realization that she had been using weight to hide from herself. One of the truths that Deidre admitted to herself regarded her sexual orientation. She realized she is a lesbian. Soon after, she ended her seventeen-year marriage with her husband, bought her own house, and met Margaret, her partner, whom she is still in love with today.

Deidre's story is not unusual to transformational nourishment. By bringing awareness to how we feed ourselves, we also have the ability to shine the light of awareness on all parts of ourselves. And then we have a choice. We can act on what we have learned to be true for ourselves, or we can look the other way. Once the layers had been shed, Deidre courageously chose to listen to the voice of her spirit and she changed her life accordingly.

By bringing awareness to what you are feeding yourself, you are in fact creating a new relationship with yourself, one in which you listen and respond to your deep needs. When a baby is born, it takes its first breaths and is soon placed on the breast. Our initial contact with the world is one of touch and nurturing. If we regard ourselves as our own ideal loving parent, we can begin to shift how we relate to ourselves, the way we talk to ourselves, how we nourish ourselves. This new relationship affects everything: all of our interpersonal relationships, our sense of work, our sense of purpose in the world. Realizing their jobs had become rote, many of my clients have made major career moves to vocations that are deeply fulfilling. Before practicing transformational nourishment, they didn't give themselves permission to listen to their true needs, let alone act on them.

Transformational nourishment provides a road map for learning how to get in touch with the place inside yourself where you are free. From that place, you can be of great service to yourself, your family, community, and to the world. Once we are willing to let go of our own limitations, we can help others do the same.

WHO ARE YOU FEEDING?

In my private practice as a nourishment consultant, I frequently ask clients the question: Who are you feeding? Sometimes *who* we are feeding is an emotion, such as happiness, or depression, sadness, and loneliness. Sometimes it is our petulant inner child who only cares about eating that candy bar right now. Or we are feeding our rebellious adolescent, who knows this particular food may not make us feel very good but goes ahead and eats it anyway, damn it! After exploring this question for themselves, nearly all of my clients discover that they have been unconsciously feeding a part of themselves that wasn't nourished. For instance, when most of us feel like we aren't being taken care of—usually when we're experiencing an emotional need—we immediately turn to the foods that were gratifying in childhood. These foods tend to be sweet, salty, or starchy.

Many people feed themselves based on an emotional need, whether the emotions are negative or positive. When people eat this way, they usually have something that's easy, fast, and requires almost no preparation. We are feeding ourselves quick fixes that usually have little nutritive value, and we're eating when we are in a state of emotional imbalance when hunger doesn't even come into the picture. Many of us are caught in old patterns of how we feed ourselves, and we don't even realize it. The question "Who are you feeding?" can be a simple antidote for this unconscious, compulsive behavior.

Let's say that you're at a party where there's a fantastic array of food. You've already eaten a delicious main course, and now a certain plate of chocolate chip cookies has attracted your attention. You saunter across the room, reach for the plate, and pop a cookie into your mouth while picking up another one. Let's pretend this is a video and we can rewind to the moment you arrive at the plate of cookies. Instead of grabbing a cookie off the plate, ask yourself our question: "Who am I feeding?" Maybe you ask your body how it would feel after you eat the cookie. You're already full from the meal, and feel the need to unbutton the top button of your pants. Is the thirty seconds of oral pleasure worth the additional discomfort to your body? Is this something you really want to do? The point isn't if you do or don't eat the cookie; the cookie itself isn't bad. The point is awareness— being aware of your actions and knowing how any particular food-stuff at any particular moment will feed you. By following the guidance and steps outlined in this book, you will learn the rhythms and needs of your body. With practice, it becomes easier to check in with yourself on a regular basis. So the next time you eat or drink something, ask yourself: "Who am I feeding?" And then wait for the honest answer.

THE JOURNEY TO NOURISHMENT

A friend of mine recently got bored with exercising in a gym and has taken to running outdoors. Running is relatively new to her and she's been informing me excitedly of the discoveries she's been making along the way. When she runs quickly and her heart rate is high, she can only last a few miles. She decided to slow down to see what would happen. By slowing her pace just a little bit, she found that she could run twice as far and with greater ease. This friend has never regarded herself as an athlete, so she is thrilled to discover she has more strength and endurance than she ever could have imagined. In this country, we're not at all used to slowing down. In fact, just about all of our modern conveniences and new technological discoveries are to help us move more quickly through life. If our lives are supposed to be easier, then why are so many people completely exhausted?

People are waking up. Our spirits are knocking, pleading to be listened to, understood, held, fed, and supported. All we have to do is open the door.

I invite you on a journey of inner growth through feeding yourself with great intention, care, and love. A true journey can't be made in a day or even in a week. Likewise, nourishment isn't a quick fix-it program; it's a slow, steady, lifetime exploration of your inner self. On this journey, there are a few rules—such as making the commitment to care for yourself—but there is no "getting it right." A Buddhist monk once told his students: "There is no good meditation; there is no bad meditation. There is just meditation." So if you fall back into addictive food patterns one day, then gently bring yourself back to center the next day. No big deal. Because transformational nourishment is *your* process, it will be uniquely your own.

Welcome to the heart of nourishment. Welcome home.

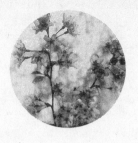

PART ONE

WHO ARE YOU FEEDING?

1

TRANSFORMATIONAL NOURISHMENT

The most visible joy can only reveal itself to us when we've transformed it, within.

—RAINER MARIA RILKE, Letters to a Young Poet

Last summer I hosted a Japanese exchange student in my home. One day we were talking about American idioms, and one that came up is "Your eyes are bigger than your stomach." My seventeen-year-old Japanese student didn't understand what this means. I asked her to take a guess. She thought a moment. "It means that what you see is more important than what you eat." Yuko's interpretation of this saying brings out an important point about how we eat: Most of us let our eyes decide what our bodies need. Our *ideas* about what we eat are more important than the food itself, what our stomachs can hold, or what we need in this moment for good, strong energy. Our families, social situations, society, and marketing campaigns dictate the choices most people make about how they feed themselves. Sometimes we're provided with very useful guidelines and models. But you need to stop and ask: Are you feeding yourself in ways that personally make sense to *your* body's unique and ever-changing needs and rhythms?

In this country, food is available all the time. Unlike our ancestors who ate in harmony with seasonal cycles of abundance and scarcity, harvest and hunting, we eat as though we're constantly feasting. Really, we eat nonstop. We fill our stomachs until we're uncomfortable, and we put more food in the shopping cart than we need. This abundance of food and our fast-paced convenience culture keep us from recognizing our own personal rhythms. We eat for many reasons, not necessarily because we're physically hungry or need certain nutrients to keep us healthy.

With more and more processed foods in the marketplace, obesity in adults and children dramatically on the rise, and digestive problems increasingly more common, it's clear that we're facing a serious health crisis. The answer, however, isn't to just put Americans on a diet. Reducing the intake of refined and processed foods and increasing fresh produce and whole grains certainly can improve one's health. But we need more. We need to feed ourselves with a sense of purpose, focus, self-love, and passion for our lives.

Now that we're in adult bodies, we can no longer rely on our mothers and fathers to fulfill our nourishment needs. Instead, we have to rely on ourselves. Although we have been feeding ourselves for many years, we still don't know what fully nourishes us. If we do recognize our hunger, then often we don't know what to eat, how much to eat, when to eat. So we guess. Our guesses at nourishment tend to lead us to familiar foods, comfort foods, convenience foods, and foods that simply don't sustain us. However, it is possible to learn what best nourishes us at any given moment.

From my friends, clients, and coworkers to my local librarian, optometrist, and cashiers at the market with whom I have a quick conversation about food, the word *nourishment* seems to always have an immediate and profound effect. Nourishment makes us look deeply into our lives. It sparks a longing for a sense of balance and wholeness, to be completely fulfilled. That's because nourishment encompasses the broad spectrum of what and how we feed ourselves to support our growth as spiritual beings. I call nourishment *transformational* because the very simple and daily act of feeding ourselves has the power to transform our lives.

People are quick to share all the ways in which they don't nourish themselves but wish they could. Deep down we intuitively know our bad habits, even if our sophisticated minds cleverly disguise them. Deep down we also know how nourishment feels—whole, safe, warm, loved, supported, energetic, clear. If we didn't have this knowledge in our gut, then I don't think so many people I've talked to over the years would have such a visceral connection to the word *nourishment*. It feels nourishing even to say the word out loud. Try it. *Nourish.* Feel how the sound escapes your mouth in the form of a deep sigh, starting with your belly and then relaxing into your entire chest.

As much as this book will explore how we nourish ourselves with food, it's important to understand that transformational nourishment is about feeding your entire being. Because the mind, body, spirit, and heart are interconnected, transformational nourishment is a circle that you can enter at any point. The key to any spiritual growth is developing awareness and responsiveness to your inner being.

I think most people would agree that we're more than just bodies mechanically walking around on earth. We're also more than minds, though where I live in the Northeast, it doesn't always seem that way! My client Sam once joked that his mind is obese. He told me that his mind has been fed too much and that he needs to feed other parts of himself that are undernourished. We use categories—physical, intellectual, emotional, and spiritual—to give us a language to talk about different realms of existence, but they are all part of the whole that makes us human. Just as our bodies are comprised of limbs, organs, and fluids that interact to form the human body, so, too, the physical, intellectual, emotional, and spiritual depend on one another to function completely. Another client, Gabrielle, put it well. "If you're selling yourself short in any one of those realms, your nourishment as a human being is incomplete." If we starve our spirits or our hearts, for instance, then we aren't nourishing ourselves to our fullest potential.

EATING VS. FEEDING

In my experience, I have found the discipline of nourishing our bodies to be an amazingly effective vehicle for spiritual development and transformation. How can food and feeding ourselves be a spiritual practice? If food seems more mundane than yoga or meditation or prayer, that's because it is. Food is one of our primary human needs. Every day, multiple times a day, we put something in our mouths. When we consume food without much thought beyond its taste, I call it *eating*. You know what eating looks like: It's the compulsive reaching into the potato chip bag; eating when you're full because food is just there; grabbing a quick bite for lunch between meetings; indulging our taste buds while ignoring how our bodies feel.

When we make deliberate food choices based on our needs for physical energy, mental clarity, creativity, and focus, I call this *feeding oneself*. I use these terms to emphasize the difference between mindless consumption and purposeful, conscious fueling. The term *feeding oneself* also shows how transformational nourishment requires two components: the part of ourselves that does the nourishing (*feeding*) and the part that receives it (*oneself*). When we feed ourselves, we are aware and responsive to our particular needs for nourishment in the present moment.

No matter how much I talk about this subject, however, it's nearly impossible to understand transformational nourishment as a theoretical approach. Transformational nourishment is profoundly practical and experiential. Because we consume food so regularly, we have the opportunity to pay attention to our inner selves multiple times a day, every day, for many years. Let's estimate that on average people feed themselves something to eat or drink fifteen times a day, though in actuality I imagine this number is a lot higher. Over a period of 10 years this translates to 54,750 opportunities to turn your attention inward and become aware of yourself. What other activity provides us with this number of chances? Not everyone meditates, or prays, or does tai chi. But feeding ourselves is something we all do, all the time.

Each morsel of food, each cup of tea is an invitation to be alert, creative, and responsive to your nourishment needs. The good news is that you can start this practice at any time. Maybe you've eaten greasy cheeseburgers, french fries, and Cokes your whole life. That's okay. It takes only one instance of consciously feeding yourself to begin the incredible journey of transformational nourishment. From the outside, that one meal may look like an ordinary plate of food, but in reality it could be the seed to a new relationship with your true self.

We've all heard the expression "you are what you eat." But what does this really mean? You eat a carrot, and you become a carrot? You eat junk food, and you become junky? While all clichés contain a grain of truth, "you are what you eat" focuses only on the after-effects of food in your body. In working with food and consciousness, I've discovered a subtle nuance to this familiar expression; that is, *people eat what they are*. If you're stressed out all the time chances are you're feeding yourself stressed-out, quick-grab foods with little vital nourishment. When we shift our way of thinking from "you are what you eat" to "you eat what you are" we see that the latter involves awareness. It makes us stop and question who we really are. If we believe that we are spiritual beings, then we're more likely to seek out the nourishing foods that feed the shining life force that already exists within us. Use this simple statement as a gentle reminder to feed yourself life-affirming foods, because you are life.

THE FACE OF NOURISHMENT

Each one of us made the journey into the world from the warm, moist, enclosed, completely supportive environment of our mother's womb. For most babies, their first contact with the physical world is to be held and nursed by their mothers. Imagine if we could remember how it felt to be held in our mother's arms, close to the same familiar heartbeat we listened to in the womb, being nourished with warm milk, totally safe and supported. Not only are babies nourished by the milk they drink, they also are fed by their close contact with people. Ideally, every baby would experience this profound and total nourishment as her or his first engagement with the physical world. If you have ever nursed or fed a baby, then you know how incredible it is to watch the baby take in the nourishment of milk. The body completely relaxes and the baby falls into a deep sleep, smiling a celestial smile. All is right with the world. This is the purest face of nourishment.

As you can see, from the earliest stage of life, feeding is much more than a physical process. When a child is hungry, she is put to the breast. When he is teething, he is fed to ease the pain. Feeding is associated with the profound nourishment of being held in loving arms, having our immediate needs met, and being connected to others.

Even if we can't remember these first precious months of life, this early connection to nourishment has been woven into the very fabric of our being. If we didn't receive this type of care in our first years, I find that almost everyone still has some early experience of being nurtured, a memory of when they felt whole, connected, and happy to be alive. A time when someone, say a grandparent or basketball coach, recognized your uniqueness and applauded your special gifts.

More and more, I hear and read the term *nourish* to describe activities that feed people emotionally, spiritually, and intellectually. I'm delighted to see this becoming more commonplace. I think of a nourishing activity as one in which you are deeply engaged in the process of life. You feel connected, empowered, creative, joyful, whole, alive. Some people may feel deeply connected to the majesty of nature while watching a sunset. Others may feel nourished sledding with their children after the first snowfall of winter, or cooking, playing the piano, taking a walk outside, or running a marathon.

When we nourish our bodies, we are feeding this same place within ourselves. Think about the times in your life when you have experienced this quality of deep fulfillment. Let these feelings be a reference for you as you learn to nourish yourself regularly through conscious food choices. The next time you find yourself engaged in a deeply nourishing activity—when you're in the heat of painting a watercolor or helping a child learn how to read—remember this feeling so you can access it later.

DINNER WITH THE UNITED NATIONS

Any time I sat down to eat, I had to check in with all of these voices in my mind to see what they wanted to eat. Who wanted to eat what, and why. There's the voice that's afraid she won't be fed, for example, and the voice that's afraid she won't be noticed. And I'm responsible for feeding all of them! Every time I sat down for a meal, it felt like I was at the United Nations. I'd have vast negotiations. But after a couple of weeks, I didn't have to do it anymore. Everyone, so to speak, knew they were going to be fed, so they could finally relax and eventually go away. Now when I sit down to a meal, I'm just feeding one person. I had been seeking this wholeness perhaps for my entire life. And now I live it. You save a lot of energy when there aren't six of you to take care of!

—GINNY

When Ginny first came to see me, she told me that food had tremendous power over her. As an example she told me she was addicted to ice cream. She had eaten it every day for many years, even during the coldest winter months. "Why do you eat it?" I asked her. "Who wants the ice cream?" I have observed in my practice that when people crave sweet, smooth dairy foods like ice cream, it sometimes relates to feelings about one's mother. This resonated for Ginny. She suddenly realized that she ate ice cream not for her present-day adult self but for the inner child that felt emotionally abandoned by her mother. Since that very day, she has almost entirely stopped eating ice cream. "I don't feel denied," she later said. "I feel freed."

I sent Ginny home from that session with a bit of homework. "When you eat this week, ask yourself *who* you're feeding." I told her that once she became familiar with asking herself *who* she's feeding, she could then pay attention to *what* she's eating, *why* she's feeding herself that particular food, and *how* she's feeding it to herself. These questions are an excellent starting point for transformational nourishment.

When we eat, we're frequently feeding ourselves from within an old emotional story. The stories vary for each of us, but they usually follow the theme of "not"—I didn't get enough love when I was a child; I'm not good enough for a lasting relationship; I don't have talent; I can't improve my health. Our pains and experiences are very real. But the stories we continually tell ourselves are masterful narratives, so masterful that we think they're the only truth.

When Ginny asked herself *who* she's feeding, she discovered a whole cast of characters: parts of herself that felt hurt, angry, lonely, frightened, undeserving of love and attention. If we try to deny these voices, they will only increase in volume. In fact, we'd be more compelled to just feed them whatever habitual comfort food they're screaming for—a dish of ice cream, a piece of pizza, doughnuts, candy, alcohol. When we feed these parts of ourselves, they only grow stronger, and at the expense of our spirit. These voices have had many years to develop persuasive personas, but we have to be gentle with our hurts. We can acknowledge our internal characters *and* choose to not feed their cravings. This is the key word: *choice.*

When you're aware of who you're feeding and why you're feeding yourself a particular food, then you have freedom to decide. You no longer are enslaved to your patterns. So if you know you're eating a bowl of chocolate ice cream because you feel rejected and lonely from a recent breakup with your partner, at least you're conscious of your choice in that moment. However, exercising this choice doesn't mean that you should spend the next hour feeling guilty and beating yourself up. The next time you find yourself reaching for the freezer door, you have another opportunity to ask yourself who you're feeding.

When my daughter came home from college for the first time, she immediately told me how much she missed eating home-cooked rice. We always have a pot on the stove, but at her college the dining hall serves overcooked and tasteless rice. So after my daughter returned to school, I was surprised to find myself suddenly wanting to eat a lot of rice. I had to stop myself. "Halé, why do you really want this? Who are you feeding?" I saw that I wasn't eating the rice for myself but for my daughter, who can't get the rice that she loves. She could eat rice three times a day. But my daughter's homesickness for rice is not *my* experience. My consuming rice certainly won't help her. All of us eat for somebody else all day long, whether it's an old part of ourselves, a loved one, or even the pain and suffering of the world. When you begin to pay attention to this dynamic, you see that in feeding these other voices, you actually miss an opportunity to nourish your true self.

Alongside the many voices seated around our United Nations dining table is one that sounds very different. This voice brings everyone to order; it is calm and aware. This voice knows exactly how we need to nourish ourselves to keep our energy strong for the next few hours, our thoughts clear, and our passions bright. Its only interest is to promote our physical, mental, emotional, and spiritual growth.

My client Alexa refers to this voice as belly wisdom. I love this expression. Most people I work with experience antagonistic relationships to their stomachs: chronic discomfort from overeating, stress, ulcers, constipation, serious digestive problems, and extra weight. At the supermarket checkout counters you can purchase any of a dozen little booklets promising you thirty days to a flat stomach. I can't help but grimace when I see or hear advertisements for drugs that will help coat people's stomachs so they can continue eating the foods that are truly damaging to their systems. In this country we're obsessed with our bellies, but in ways that prevent us from hearing its wisdom.

"When I need to make decisions, I turn to my stomach," explains Alexa. "When I really want to know my truth—how I feel about a person, how I feel about my job, even what I should have for dinner—I listen to my belly wisdom. Then I have no doubt about my decisions. There's a clear line between my head and my belly." When we have a deep feeling about something, we say that we know it in our gut or that it's a gut instinct. When we nourish ourselves attentively and lovingly with vital foods, we clear out the physical and emotional debris in our systems, allowing us to access this place of internal wisdom. The cleanse, which is explained in chapter 5, is an excellent way to get a taste of how this works.

As we've talked about, people have the tendency to feed their emotions. Alexa also acknowledges this tendency in herself. "When I'm stressed out, depressed, or tired," she told me, "my inclination is to feed those emotions. Or I'll want to celebrate when I feel happy with ice cream or pretzels or M&M's. When I was in graduate school and studying very intensely, I depended on sugar and carbohydrates to keep me going. Then I saw that if I ate almonds or walnuts instead, I was feeding my brain rather than my empty spaces. I learned how to feed my wholeness. I had to let go of how society and my family have always told me I should eat and discover what was right for me."

KINDNESS STARTS AT HOME:
LEARNING TO RECEIVE

When you're nourished, you are fulfilled. You feel a pervasive sense of well-being. And it's enough. How often do we really let ourselves feel that something is enough? Earlier in this chapter we talked about the term *feeding oneself* and how nourishment requires both giving and receiving. The giving part of nourishment is easy to recognize—a fresh salad, homemade soup, grilled vegetables. The receiving is where we come to a screeching halt. I know generous and loving people who give so much to their families and friends yet have a very difficult time receiving from others—including themselves.

We cannot be nourished if we don't allow ourselves to receive. To receive nourishment, we need to be open. Yes, we open our mouths to take in food, but that's about all we're receiving most of the time. Transformational nourishment means that our bodies, hearts, minds, and spirits are open and willing to take in the nourishment that's offered. To do this, we have to believe that we are valuable and worthy to receive.

Why is it so difficult for us to embrace ourselves for who we are? Psychologically, each one of us has our own negative story of how we didn't get what we needed in life, particularly in our youth. In turn, we become paralyzed. What paralyzes us isn't the actual neglect, abuse, or other painful experience, but the negative story itself. We repeatedly tell ourselves the story of how our needs won't be met, and we assume crash position to protect ourselves. Because this belief is so strong, we ultimately create patterns that in fact don't meet our needs. We eat fast food, junk food, eat on the run or while reading e-mail and listening to phone messages, and don't give ourselves the time and space that will support our well-being. It becomes a self-fulfilling cycle: I don't believe my deep needs will be met, so I create a lifestyle where they can't possibly be fulfilled. In the end, we create exactly what we're fighting against!

I never ask people to negate these stories. I think that's a real recipe for disaster because the negative stories will only get stronger. Instead, I encourage people to be curious about the moments of wholeness in their lives, the times of genuine happiness when their needs were fulfilled. And it was enough. From that one tiny seed—the ten minutes of watching snow fall, the hour with a favorite uncle, dancing, being enraptured by music, playing in the park with your golden retriever—we can germinate an entire life of connection, purpose, and well-being. If your internal radio has been set to one negative station for a long time, then why not try turning the dial to see what else your receiver can pick up. Trust me, there is another station. It may come in faintly at first, maybe even with some static. But the voice of your spirit is always present. To hear it, you simply have to be willing to receive.

But what does it mean to be receptive? On the one hand, we already know it has to do with an attitude of openness. If receptivity is open, it equally must be discerning. What are we willing to receive and how much? The illusion of receptivity is that we're available to everybody and everything at all times. Our door is always open. But that's not true receptivity. True receptivity is clear about boundaries: We know where our needs begin and end. In fact, the more receptive and sensitive you become, the more selective you must be about what you are willing to receive.

We can learn from our own body's biology. Each one of our cells selectively feeds, knowing exactly what it needs to take in for nourishment. The wall of the cell opens to receive nutrients or to eliminate waste, and then it closes again. The innate wisdom of the body knows how to maintain balance and wholeness at all times, beginning with this fundamental activity of the cell. Like the very cells that comprise our bodies, we too have the ability to know how to selectively feed ourselves only that which serves us best. At the molecular level this pattern already exists within us. All we have to do is go along with our own natural rhythm. The information in part 2 of this book offers practical suggestions for becoming more discerning about what you take in to your physical, emotional, and spiritual body. Through regular practice, we can learn how to become clear about everything we select to consume—from foods to media, movies, books, and conversations.

People frequently use the expression "my plate is too full" to mean they are swamped with work and other life responsibilities and can't possibly handle any more. I would take the metaphor a step further. Not only are our plates too full, our bodies are too full, our minds are too full, our houses and calendars and just about everything else in our lives are too full. Most people eat with the TV or radio on, in the car, reading the paper, at the office while working on the computer, while rushing between meetings or errands and carpools. With so much external stimulation, how can we possibly pay attention to what we're feeding ourselves? We grab whatever is readily available and eat as though every meal is our last. In reality, this translates into perpetual feasting. This excess creates confusion. Anytime there's excess, we can't think straight, feel straight, or know what kind of nourishment we need to receive from moment to moment. To receive nourishment, we need to make space, and making space means perpetually letting go of that which is no longer necessary.

If we are present and loving when we feed ourselves just one meal in the course of a day or a week, then a remarkable thing happens. We eat less because we receive more. It's very subtle. Each time we feed ourselves is an opportunity to connect to our bodies, our hearts, our minds, our spirits. Right here. Right now. In this moment.

2

THE WAKE-UP CALL

Moyers: Do you ever have this sense when you are following your bliss, as I have at moments, of being helped by hidden hands?

Campbell: All the time. It is miraculous. I even have a superstition that has grown on me as the result of invisible hands coming all the time—namely, that if you do follow your bliss you put yourself on a kind of track that has been there all the while, waiting for you, and the life that you ought to be living is the one you are living. When you can see that, you begin to meet people who are in the field of your bliss, and they open the doors to you. I say, follow your bliss and don't be afraid, and doors will open where you didn't know they were going to be.

—JOSEPH CAMPBELL WITH BILL MOYERS, The Power of Myth

BETH'S STORY

I believe we're always getting called to wake up and make changes in our lives, if only we can listen. I heard the call, but I ignored it. I knew that I needed to leave my job and completely restructure my life, but I was afraid. The call came again, and I still didn't listen. I'm a pretty stubborn person. And then I got cancer. Now I no longer had the luxury to ignore my spirit, which had been begging me to pay attention to my life.

For several years I had the gnawing feeling that something was wrong, but I just couldn't put my finger on it. I was a partner at a high-powered law firm, where I had worked for nearly twenty years. My job had grown to be much more than one person could handle, and it took all my energy. I didn't have the time or strength to care properly for my daughter, my husband, or myself. Eventually, the stress in my life began to take its toll on my health. In a five-year period, I had three years of infertility, my gall bladder was removed, and I experienced debilitating back pain. I knew I was unhappy but I wasn't listening, even to the signs of my body.

I would tell my friends that I was in a hole, and I didn't know how to climb out. I said, "If I don't do something about my life, my body will do it for me."

Looking for ways to cope, I tried yoga and visited healers. One woman said to me, "Your environment doesn't work for you. You want to go home. You really want to go home." What did this mean? I wasn't domestic at all. Cooking for me consisted of heating up a can of SpaghettiOs. I quickly dismissed her words. Now I see that she couldn't have been more right. I did want to go home; I desperately wanted to come home to myself.

But the thought of change, of leaving the only job I have ever known, left me panic-stricken: Who would I be? What would I do with my life? And how would I ever get my husband to support my leaving such a lucrative position without any financially viable plan for the future? Yet I knew that I absolutely needed time off, something more substantial than our yearly vacations. After months of telling myself I would never be able to get the time I wanted, I finally found the courage to try to make a change. I asked my boss if I could reduce my schedule to three days a week and, more importantly, hire someone full-time to take over part of my responsibilities. To my surprise and delight, he said yes. It was so simple. After all the anxiety and inner turmoil, once I decided to change my lifestyle, all I had to do was ask for what I needed.

Ironically, within weeks of this decision and just when I started to feel better than I had in a long time, I found blood in my stool one evening.

That same week I happened to visit my doctor for a regular physical. I didn't really think much about the blood, but I decided to mention it. The next day I left my office for a colonoscopy, not knowing that I wouldn't return to my desk for another nine months. Two days later, surgeons removed almost two feet of my colon. The cancer was an aggressive form and the tumor had already broken through the colon wall. Miraculously, the cancer hadn't yet spread to other parts of my body. The doctors were shocked that I had been functioning at all, let alone without more symptoms than a few traces of blood.

I longed to get out of my busy, stressful life, and I did—though not necessarily in the way that I had wanted or imagined. There's nothing easy about cancer, but I tell you those nine months were the best time of my adult life. I had never felt so peaceful or happy, so free from my own and others' expectations of how and what I was supposed to be. I wrote songs, filled journal after journal. For the first time, I could contemplate my life and make yoga, meditation, and nutrition a regular part of my day. I called this my own internal chemotherapy; even if a bad cell had escaped, I could still heal and strengthen my body and my spirit.

In the course of my recovery, I rediscovered a vital part of myself, a part of me that I hadn't felt since I was very young. I tapped into my creativity and insight, the place within myself where there's no fear. A friend of mine once said to me, "I would hate to live inside your head." I used to be so filled with fear and insecurity all the time, but this person I discovered wasn't afraid at all. I completely trusted my healing; I felt that I was being carried by the universe. Even during my chemotherapy treatments, I felt like blessings were raining down on me.

I had been called to come home, but I needed to find a way to get there. All the chemo in the world wouldn't fix me if I couldn't be at home in my body. I eventually realized that there's a place inside us of perfect peace, clarity, joy, and balance. It's always there; we don't even have to seek it out. I stayed in this place for nine months. Most of us just don't know how to find our way back to it. My chief lesson was remembering that this place exists and learning how to honor this part of myself without having to get sick to do it.

The call isn't a one-shot deal. I eventually returned to my job, but found myself crying for months. Before, I simply knew that something was wrong in my life. Now I also knew that I was being called to a whole new way of life and that my heart and soul were elsewhere. During those nine precious months, I had discovered that my true vocation in life is to help others by sharing the lessons of my own dramatic healing. But my husband still didn't think we could afford to lose my law firm salary. That spring I told the women in my cleanse group that I had the feeling I would be able to leave my firm that summer. The minute I said it, I knew there was no turning back. I didn't even tell my family about this knowing, but every day I would remind myself of my intention to return to the life I had found. One afternoon in June, completely out of the blue, my husband called me at work. "Okay, you can retire," he said. "We'll be fine."

I've been home now for a few months, cooking nourishing meals for my family, completing a yoga teacher training program, and meditating so I can tune in regularly to my inner voice. My family can't believe how peaceful and happy I am. I truly believe that the cancer saved my life, though I wouldn't wish for anyone to travel the same life-threatening road I took to finally wake up to my spiritual path. The call is ringing again. I feel that I am being called to help others discover inner balance, particularly individuals in the corporate environment who struggle so much with work and life balance at the expense of their own physical, mental, and spiritual well-being. There's work to do, but it hasn't yet begun. I need to remind myself that I don't have to know exactly what's next. I'm getting really good at trusting this not-knowing. It makes everything possible.

COMING HOME TO YOUR SPIRIT

Embedded within each of us is our own particular spiritual call. The call is a reminder that we are spiritual beings, with our own unique gifts and contributions to offer on earth. Nearly every religious tradition agrees that one of our chief purposes in life is to help others. In my terminology, I like to say that we are instruments of transformation and change. To be of service, we need to nourish ourselves. Only then can we learn how best to serve others, to ultimately benefit the world.

Ecologists use the metaphor of a web to demonstrate how all life is interconnected and how our actions in one place can affect the environment in another location thousands of miles away. The calling, which sounds from the time we are born, is an inducement to realize your true self, and your place in the web of life. Just as each of us has a unique fingerprint, so, too, we have our own particular gifts to share with the world. The call is the clarion voice of your spirit telling you, dear reader, that you are precious and that your presence here on earth is valuable to the welfare of the entire world.

Transformational nourishment is a practice to help you continually respond to your calling. It trains and strengthens us to listen to the subtle messages of our inner guidance. There are many ways to strengthen ourselves to be of greater service to the world: prayer, meditation, yoga, tai chi, Qigong, nourishment through food practices, and other healing arts. The Dalai Lama once commented on how wonderful it is that so many different spiritual practices exist to suit all the different varieties of human personality. For most people, committing to one or two of these practices usually is enough to learn how to live a spiritual life, a life in which our spirit is infused in all our activities. It's good to follow a practice that deeply engages and inspires you, but you certainly don't need to practice everything all at once. If you were drawn to transformational nourishment, then you likely feel connected to the daily act of feeding yourself as a practice for spiritual growth.

How do we know when we're being called? The actual form of the call is entirely unique to each individual, and depends on what is needed to get your attention. While the call is always ringing and available for us to answer, we're normally just not willing to listen. Unfortunately, it sometimes takes poor health, hitting an emotional low, feeling dissatisfied with work, having trouble with a relationship, or another major life problem to bring us to the point where we have no choice but to listen to the call.

Regardless of the particular form the call may take, the purpose is always the same: You are being called to wake up and come home to your spiritual essence, to the person you really are. Like Beth, many of the clients I have seen over the years have expressed a profound desire to go home. They long to connect to the part of themselves that is whole, balanced, wise, and discerning of life's true priorities. Ultimately, the call demands that we change. We're asked—though sometimes it feels more like pushed—to let go of the narrow ways in which we've perceived ourselves so that we can live in true freedom.

THE CALL TO WAKE UP

Have you ever noticed how some people are "morning people," while others are better left alone until after noon? I'm the kind of person who can wake up easily in the morning. I love the early hours, when the house is still quiet and I can have time alone to meditate, read, drink a cup of tea, putter in my garden during the warm months. My daughter is just the opposite. She likes to stay up until all hours of the night, so she has a hard time getting up early. It was particularly challenging to get her out of bed when she was in high school and had to be in class at 7:30 in the morning. Because she frequently slept through the alarm, she got in the habit of setting at least three clocks. From nearly everywhere in the house, you could hear the high-pitched buzz starting at 6:30 A.M. Yasemin would then hit the snooze button—what an invention!— and go back to sleep. Eight minutes later, again the alarms would drone their mechanical beeps. Snooze. Buzz. Snooze. Buzz. Eventually, she would drag herself out of bed, sometimes with a little encouragement from her father or me.

The call is like our own internal alarm clock. It's a wake-up call from our spirit to pay attention to our lives. To ask ourselves the big questions: Who am I? Why am I here? How can I live a truly rewarding life? Sometimes the alarm buzzes and we can respond immediately. Other times, we hit snooze. When that happens, the call will come again—perhaps not eight minutes later as with my daughter's clocks, but you can definitely count on it buzzing again sometime in the future.

At some point in our lives, each one of us will be called to wake up. By *waking up* I mean the profound realization that we are spiritual beings and that we must respect and nourish all parts of ourselves with that awareness. You are being called on the greatest journey that exists: to explore the inner regions of yourself. The best part is that you don't have to plan, research, or pay a cent for this trip. You don't have to *do* anything to book your passage. The call will come on its own. All you need to do is *allow* yourself to listen.

Maybe you're thinking, "Gee, receiving your own personal call would be great, but nothing like that ever happens to me. I'm just an ordinary person. What happens if I don't get called?" You can even imagine your spirit shrugging its shoulders and saying, "Oh well, I guess you missed your chance. Better luck next time."

David Spangler addresses this concern in *The Call*, a book entirely devoted to the subject of the spiritual calling. "What happens if I never get a call? Well, that doesn't happen," Spangler says. "We are always called. . . . But I may never hear a voice or see an angel telling me what to do. I may never feel some force overwhelming my life and sending me forth on a quest or mission. I may never have some specific experience that tells me, 'This is your identity. This is your destiny.' The challenge, then, is, can I see past the lack of such phenomena to realize that I've already gotten, and have always gotten, the primal call?" As Spangler indicates, the magic of the call is that it isn't an extraordinary event in the lives of lucky or special people. I assure you that there's nothing exceptional about the call. This is very important to understand. The call happens in ordinary people's lives, and it will happen in yours. If you were interested in reading this book, your own calling just may be ringing right now.

Many of my clients hear the call when they're in the midst of a life transition. Beginning or ending a relationship. Switching jobs or careers. Moving. Retiring. Completing a degree. Having children. The children leaving home. These transitions are important for us to pay attention to. They provide enough of a gap in our identity—we're in the process of changing from who we were to who we're becoming—to get us to pay attention to our inner life. These moments are ripe for hearing the wake-up call. Suddenly you realize that you're not just mourning the death of your mother but that you are reconnecting with your own forgotten sense of self and purpose.

If we miss the quieter inklings of the wake-up call, then the call finds more dramatic ways to get our attention, as it did with Beth. Many of my clients first come to see me with physical complaints. Their bodies feel out of balance, and they are looking for a way to regain health, vitality, and a sense of well-being. I've worked with clients who have cancer, fibromyalgia, TMJ, Crohn's disease, acid reflux, irritable bowel syndrome, headaches, severe PMS, eczema, and weight problems. These physical disturbances usually don't develop overnight. By the time the client is sitting on the sofa across from me, his or her body has most likely been out of balance for quite some time. For these clients, their bodies are relaying the message of the call. The body says, "We've done it your way long enough. I've had it. It's time to learn how to take care of yourself." In regaining health, we need patience. We need to realize that the human being is a whole system and that healing the body also involves the spirit, heart, and mind. Healing doesn't occur in a day, with a few herbs and vitamins, or a soy shake. Instead, the wake-up call informs us, we must make nourishing ourselves a priority and commit to a daily practice of caring for ourselves on all levels.

When Yolanda became my client, she was about to hit rock bottom. At twenty-three, she was exhausted, depressed, and on Prozac. After graduating from college, she worked in finance and went out to clubs and bars almost every night of the week. This lifestyle was quickly burning her out, and she knew it. Still, she had the idea that this is how a twenty-something-year-old should live, and, besides, it was easier to go along with the crowd. Everyone else seemed to be having fun, but a voice within Yolanda kept insisting she wasn't being true to herself, and that there was more to life.

Yolanda heard this voice and she listened. I admire her for responding to the call at an already challenging time in life when people are claiming their independence and defining themselves personally and professionally. Yolanda's call required her to go against the grain, to stop blindly following the crowd. For the first time in her adult life, she began to spend time alone, and stopped rushing wildly from one extreme to another. She realized her life was hers to create, and that she didn't have to go along with the crowd. "Starting with the basics of food, I began applying what I learned to other areas of my life," she said. "What are my basic needs? Rest. Time for myself. More quiet. I make sure these needs are met first before I do anything else. It's constant work. I take one step forward and two steps back. But I notice how I'm changing and growing. I look to myself for answers, and I know that my internal wisdom is there if I choose to listen. When I do listen, it always works out."

Deep down we fear that answering the call means giving up our lives. We fear we will lose ourselves. And it's true; you do have to make a sacrifice. What you sacrifice is who you are *not*: the false perceptions about yourself and how you've been living. Eventually, this comes as a great relief. It takes much more energy to deceive yourself about your true happiness than it does to simply let go and be yourself. A client once described this as trying to hold up a steel wall with your hands coated in grease. "Why don't you just let go of the wall?" I asked him. He looked at me dumbfounded. He had never considered this possibility before.

As humans, we have great resistance to change. So we hide from the call. We pull the blankets over our heads and believe that nobody can see us. The more we resist the call, the more life feels like a struggle. I've seen this over and over again. People feel isolated and overburdened by how much energy it takes to maintain the old form. The wake-up call begs us to stop living on autopilot and to take real responsibility for nourishing our authentic selves. Life constantly presents us with the surprises and circumstances that demand us to change. If our bodies don't regularly change, then we would not be alive. The same is true for our spiritual, emotional, and intellectual lives. The wake-up call invites us to be flexible and to dance with life. When we start responding, even in a timid way, we see the call's inherent goodness. We begin to understand that while change and letting go are difficult, we're only being challenged to become who we really are.

THE CALL TO RECONNECT

The summer before my senior year of high school, my family moved from Wisconsin to the Washington, D.C., area. When I started school that fall, I didn't know a single person. I was in shock. For the second time since I immigrated at age eight, my entire world had turned upside down. I had lost all my friends. I was seventeen and struggling to separate my identity from my overprotective Turkish family. I felt like an outsider in my town, school, and family. As difficult and lonely as this time in my life was, it proved to be the best thing that could have happened to me. My sudden position as an outsider forced me to rely on myself in a whole new way, and I began to ask myself questions about life's meaning and true happiness.

My inner inquiry continued when I went to college. It was the late 1960s, and the times were ripe for those of us seeking to develop our consciousness. Once I got started on this path, there was no holding me back. I became deeply inquisitive about spiritual practices and began reading yoga scriptures and accounts of holy people who had worked with their bodies as instruments for spiritual growth. My quest wasn't just an intellectual exercise. I practiced yoga; prepared and fed myself whole foods; and studied Hinduism, Buddhism, Sufism, and mystical Christianity. My instincts told me that deep fulfillment only comes by looking within and making a connection to our spirit. I ached for this connection, to finally feel that I was coming home to myself.

"The territory of the self is a vast, unexplored, and prohibited geography," writes the author Deena Metzger. She continues: ". . . our experiences, feelings, insights, understandings are often off-limits. As often as we are imprisoned inside ourselves, so often are we actually living in exile outside ourselves. One can say that one of the basic conditions of contemporary life is the unfulfilled longing of the self for itself."

I think the word *exile* is very interesting in this context. To live in exile means one has an original homeland. One knows the experience of home. If we think about ourselves living in exile outside of ourselves, then we begin to see that we already know what it feels, looks, and sounds like to be home. If you have ever experienced homesickness—at overnight camp or your first year in college or living abroad—then you know how missing home can feel like an empty hole in your stomach. This longing is good. It's the essential motivator to begin the process of returning home, of reconnecting to all aspects of yourself. While we may feel as though we are in exile, the truth is that someone has been home the entire time. That someone is your spirit. The call is your spirit's way of beckoning you on the journey home.

My client Khandro once told me that she used to eat as though she were a tourist on vacation. "The way I eat," she told me during one of our first sessions, "I treat myself like a crappy tourist with a box lunch. I tell myself I'll start eating right tomorrow because then I'll be home. But I'm never home!" Khandro is a professor, and her demanding schedule keeps her busy and away from home for long hours each day. Like many people, Khandro was in the habit of eating on the go, grabbing food at the college cafeteria, eating junk food between classes, and indulging in cheese platters, pastries, trays of cookies, and all the other "free food" at meetings and conferences. Before she began to work with me, Khandro didn't know one vegetable from the next because she never cooked for herself. When I asked her what it means to eat at home compared to the tourist mode, she said, "Eating at home means someone loves me and I belong."

When I see a client for the first time, we sit down and have a cup of tea together and talk. We usually talk for several hours. During this first session, I ask everyone the same question: Can you remember a time in your life when you felt whole, connected, at home within yourself? Without fail, every person I have asked has been able to remember at least one experience, perhaps one small moment, of wholeness. It can take many tears for people to find their experience, to journey back through all the layers of protection and hurt and disappointment to finally remember the night when they watched snow falling in the streetlamp outside their bedroom window and had the overwhelming feeling of being connected to each snowflake, and the wind, and the orange halo of light around the lamp. At the time, this particular client was a suicidal teenager struggling with the twin feelings of isolation and despair. The beauty of the snow inspired her to write a poem, and then another poem. She is now a poet. Moments of wholeness tend to be those when we feel vital, balanced, and connected—to our loved ones or other people, to ourselves, to the earth, to creative energy, to the source of all life. Wholeness is the opposite of isolation. The voice of isolation whispers: "What's the use?" The voice of connection says: "You, the person holding this book in your hands right now, *you matter*."

THE CALL TO TRANSFORM

It would be nice if we could go to sleep one night as our regular tired, aching, cranky, dispassionate selves and wake up in the morning bright, eager, vivacious, with a permanent sense of well-being coursing from the tops of our heads to our toes. But transformation doesn't happen overnight. I don't know of any elixir that can produce the real changes in health, awareness, and well-being that people so desperately desire except for the steady discipline and commitment to nourishing ourselves.

Transformation is the most awesome and awe-inspiring part about being human. Transformation allows us to shed our skin over and over again. If we hear and respond to the call, then we already have triggered the process of transforming ourselves. How will we be transformed? What will our new selves look like? The mind agitates for answers, clear goals, an assurance of logical results. Of course, it's easier to agree to something if we know what the outcome will be. As much as we can know with our intellect that growth is an essential component of life and our development as human beings, transformation equally requires our trust and faith in the unknown.

I read a wonderful commentary by Rabbi Sheffa Gold on the biblical story of Exodus, when the Israelites realize that they are slaves and must leave their bondage in Egypt. "First there's leaving Egypt," she says in an interview quoted in the book *The Cultural Creatives*. "Which means that you realize that you're caught. And then you hear a call. Something pushes you out, wakes you up, makes you realize what slavery is." Of course, the Exodus story continues to dramatically unfold with the Israelites fleeing toward freedom. Discussing the moment when the Israelites arrive at the Red Sea with the Egyptian army breathing down their backs, Rabbi Gold cites an interesting point from the midrash, a rabbinical story. According to the midrash, the Red Sea didn't part until a man named Nachson walked into the sea up to his nose. Rabbi Gold goes on to explain this peculiar detail. "What mattered was his faith . . . and also knowing that there wasn't anything else to do. When the forces of the old life are behind you, and the sea is ahead of you, the waters aren't going to part unless somebody starts walking."

Responding to the call means letting go of the old in order to create room for new growth. That's not to say that you have to let go of everything, or suddenly develop amnesia and forget where you've come from. In the process of letting go, we sometimes feel as though the earth has been pulled out from beneath us and we're suspended in midair. The old structure is falling away, and the new one has yet to appear. This is where faith becomes critical. If the Israelites knew that they would wander in a desert for the next forty years, I imagine they wouldn't have been terribly inclined to leave the comfort and familiarity of their old lives, even though they were slaves and the wandering eventually led to their true liberation.

Because we don't have any guarantees of the new life, we have to trust the wisdom of our spirit to guide us into the next stage of growth. Whether it's leaving an unfulfilling relationship, a dissatisfying career, or the bondage of biblical Egypt, the call will always take us from a limiting perspective of one's life into the expansive field of living according to the essence and direction of one's spirit. When you feel the call so strongly that you *know* you are made of spirit, then like Nachson you won't hesitate to step into the water. You will be willing to say yes. We struggle so hard with change, even when we know it's for our highest good, that when we do finally accept the call, it comes as a wave of relief. We can surrender our illusions that we are all alone in the world. In entering the water, there's a sense of losing our small self. But that's exactly what we've wanted for a long time, to align with our spirit self.

When you're looking into the face of the unknown, of course it's natural to feel fear. Just as snakes regularly shed their skins, so, too, we transform periodically throughout our lives. When we can witness ourselves in the act of shedding our skin a few times, we begin to trust our spirit more. Eventually, this trust becomes rock solid. With experience comes the faith and understanding that your spirit always directs you to the next stage necessary for your growth. When you are in the midst of a transformational moment in your life, you may not necessarily understand exactly where your spirit is leading you; you don't even have to like it. But you do have to trust it. I can assure you that your spirit will never steer you wrong. Never.

The transformative process is the most profound aspect of responding to the call because, as we've talked about, change is not an overnight process. We have a relationship with our spiritual, psychological, emotional, and physical development. We dance with it. We cry with it. Sometimes it's not easy. In fact, most of the time it's a challenge. Nourishment means shaking the sleep out of your eyes and being awake on a regular basis. As we grow, so, too, does our confidence in our ability to nourish our spirit. We learn that we can always rely on our spirit for stability as we wander the unfamiliar and sometimes uncomfortable parts of ourselves on the journey toward balance and well-being.

3

EMBODYING SPIRIT

*If I am not for myself, then who will be for me? And if I am
only for myself, then what am I? And if not now, when?*

—RABBI HILLEL, *first century* C.E.

Why are we really here? It's a good question, don't you think?
I think so, too; that's why I asked a group of college students to
answer it. The depth and sincerity of their answers impressed me.
This is what they had to say: *To be of service. To wake up. To teach. To
enjoy everything. To learn. To be connected. To discover and use our gifts. To
understand love.*

All of these answers are true, of course. However, when I
asked the students this question, I wasn't looking for a particular
answer. The main thing wasn't their answers but the thinking that
the question would provoke. Maybe you remember staying up all
night in college debating the big questions of life, as I did when I
was a student in the 1960s. Or perhaps you came to these questions
only later in life, or they are just now starting to dance on the edges
of your mind and heart. Who am I? What's the meaning of life?
Why am I really here?

These questions are not sophomoric musings. They are
essential and good. It's the big questions that inspire profound discoveries, creativity, and self-inquiry. Unless we explore the deep
questions about the meaning and purpose of life, the idea of nourishing yourself as a spiritual being won't make a lot of sense. Intro-

spection is essential to transformational nourishment because this work isn't just about making dietary changes; it's about a change of consciousness. No matter how many of the right foods you feed yourself from the suggestions in this book, this is just another set of guidelines if you aren't willing to do the work of self-awareness. We're not talking about losing a few pounds here; we're talking about serious transformation!

It's okay if we don't have all the answers to the meaning of life. It takes courage to ask the difficult questions and even more valor to admit when we don't know, and to remain steady in that place of unknowing. In the famous correspondence between the master poet and the poet just learning his craft, Rainer Maria Rilke wisely counsels the young Mr. Kappus "to be patient toward all that is unsolved in your heart and to try to love the *questions themselves* like locked rooms and like books that are written in a very foreign tongue. Do not now seek the answers, which cannot be given you because you would not be able to live them. And the point is, to live everything. *Live* the questions now. Perhaps you will then gradually, without noticing it, live along some distant day into the answer."

As Westerners, we're privileged with abundant educational and financial resources, and the ability to exert a lot of influence in the world. We can read spiritual books like this one and consider our lives from many different perspectives beyond the meeting of our basic daily needs. For this very reason we have a responsibility to wake up and be of greater service in the world. With nourishment, I have seen over and over again that if we feed ourselves with intention and love, and with life-filled foods, our everyday lives become more infused with spirit and spiritual direction. It's no longer just about getting up in the morning, going to work, coming home, and going to bed. The daily routine still exists, but every aspect of life is infused with a greater purpose.

BECOMING A STRONG VEHICLE FOR SPIRIT

Imagine for a moment that you've just purchased a new house. After you move in, the first heavy rain reveals that you have a leaky roof. For the interior to remain beautiful and undamaged, the exterior also must be solid. The same is true for us. We need to make our bodies into strong physical containers for our spirits to grow, expand, and be more present in our lives. The stronger the physical container, the more vibrant our spirits will be; the stronger the spirit, the more we naturally want to strengthen the body.

By "strong" physical container, I don't mean that you have to suddenly start weight training or take up kickboxing. Bodies come in all different types, sizes, and abilities. In this context, strength has to do with nourishing your own wonderful unique self to your most optimum, not an Olympic athlete's. Remember, transformational nourishment isn't necessarily about obtaining your ideal physical shape. We strengthen ourselves to stay physically balanced and energetically supple so that we can listen to our spirit's messages. The more vibrant and sensitive our bodies are, the easier it is for spirit to work through us. If the body isn't balanced, it's more difficult to feel your spirit. Certainly it's possible, but physical distress consumes a lot of attention and energy. A common cold is enough to sap us of our energy, let alone the chronic distresses of headaches, gastrointestinal problems, rashes, and allergies.

We desire deeper meaning and purpose in our lives, but to achieve this we have to be willing to do the work. In our goal-oriented minds, we believe that if we work hard enough, one day we will finally arrive at our own brand of utopia: perfect health, perfect relationship, perfect profession, perfect family, perfect happiness. Not only are we fixated on these goals, we're also impatient. How many times on long car trips do your kids repeatedly ask the familiar question: "Are we there yet?" I know our kids annoyed us plenty of times from the backseat of the car. Regardless if we had five or fifty miles left to go, the response was always the same: "We'll get there when we get there." In other words, there's no way to speed up the process. The journey is everything.

The practice of consciously feeding yourself sets awareness into motion. Awareness isn't something that you keep in a box and use only for certain parts of your life. It's all-encompassing. Awareness of your physical nourishment leads to awareness of yourself emotionally and spiritually. This is how awareness works. If you shine a flashlight in a dark room, only a small portion of the room will light up, right? From this limited view, you wouldn't know how big the room was or everything that it contained. But if you switched on the ceiling light, you'd suddenly see the room in its entirety, with its marvelous furnishings, oil paintings, and Turkish rugs.

Awareness is like the ceiling light: It has the power to illuminate all parts of yourself. The more you nourish yourself, the stronger the wattage of your awareness becomes. Spiritual growth arises out of regular, daily practice. If you've felt called to wake up and listen to your spirit, then make the commitment to feed this part of your life. The seed of your spiritual self is already planted in fertile soil; all you have to do is nourish it. Take heart. As Lao Tzu says in the *Tao Te Ching*, "What is rooted is easy to nourish."

JOSEF'S STORY

The morning of June 6, 1986, I woke up, dressed, made breakfast, got the older children off to school, and began my day. I can't remember what happened next because it was just another day, like all the other ordinary days that had come before it. I couldn't have known that all my strengths, beliefs, intuitive abilities, the very fabric of my marriage and community, and everything I had learned about nourishment and healing would soon be tested.

It was Friday afternoon, my turn to carpool the kids home from school. My oldest son, Micah, middle son, Josef, and Jesse, one of their close friends, were jabbering away about whatever happened to be the latest and greatest of the moment. It had started to rain. As we were approaching an intersection, a truck ran a stop sign and plowed into the rear passenger side of the car, where six-year-old Josef was buckled into his car seat. The car spun around 360 degrees before finally crashing into a telephone pole on the opposite side of the street. Our car was totaled. The seventeen-year-old driver of the truck walked away without a scratch. Micah and Jesse had cuts and scrapes all over their bodies, but I wasn't hurt at all. I quickly realized when I saw Josef that he had taken the brunt of the impact. When I saw my son, he was bloody and unconscious.

All I knew was that I had to get Josef out of the car. Because of the impact, the passenger door wouldn't open. You've probably heard stories about ordinary people who suddenly acquire heroic strength to rescue somebody. I can tell you it's true. Josef was a hefty child, but somehow I managed to pull his heavy, limp body out through the smashed-in, glassless window. I laid him on the grass and checked to see if he was breathing. Miraculously, he was. Someone called an ambulance. When we arrived at the local hospital, the critical nature of Josef's condition was apparent and we were transferred to a large Boston hospital, where he underwent a seven-hour surgery that night.

When someone suffers brain damage as extensively as our son did, chances of survival are low. The chances of living and not being vegetative are even rarer. So we were told by the doctors. The top neurologists told us that Josef was not likely to survive because of the severe pressure in his brain. If he did survive, he would be vegetative for the rest of his life, at best. If we believed the doctors, I'm convinced that Josef would have remained vegetative. But we listened to our son, and he knew he was going to fully recover.

Three days after the accident, Josef was still in a coma. His condition had worsened and the doctors told us there was a chance he wouldn't survive through the night. I stayed home with my other children while Steven, my husband, and a minyan of men gathered at the hospital to pray at Josef's bedside. In the middle of the night, I woke up and heard a train in the distance. I understood that there was a crossing over. I knew with the depth of my being that Josef was making the decision to live or die, not as a six-year-old boy but as a spiritual being choosing life or death. As a mother, I would have been utterly devastated to lose my son. Yet I also knew that this was beyond the realm of mother and son. That night I communicated with my son's spirit. I let him know that I would be totally committed to him if he wished to come back and that I also would be willing to let him go if he needed to leave. I gave him free choice to act as his spirit needed. Steven later told me that he had conveyed the same message to our son.

Josef lived through the night. Still, the doctors prepared us for the worst. Soon after, I was nursing my daughter at home when I suddenly felt Josef's presence in her room. "I'm coming back, Mama," I heard him say. That was all the confirmation I needed. I told him I would do everything in my power to bring him back to health. Our son had made a commitment, and so had I. I knew then, as I do now, that for Josef to survive the accident not just as a body but as a vibrant and vital *person*, means that our son has an extraordinarily strong spirit. "I'm coming back, Mama" showed that his spirit still had work to do in this lifetime. I didn't have grand ideas about the person that our son would grow up to be or what he would do with his life. As his mother and fellow spiritual being, I made the commitment to support him unconditionally, no matter the challenges ahead. In time we would all learn that an accident isn't a one-time crisis but a long series of collisions: Josef's healing, our family's healing, would take a lifetime.

It took great strength, vision, and commitment to work with this limp body that had been given up for dead and could be only vegetative and nothing else. I had to rely on all of my resources to help bring Josef back to his fullest capabilities. Sometimes this took me on a very different route than what the medical field was suggesting. Some of these approaches have become more common today, but in the 1980s this was not the norm. Josef remained in a coma for a month. During those weeks, my husband and I spent twelve hours a day, every day, encouraging Josef to regain consciousness. We showered him with love and support, reading his favorite books and talking to him although he was unconscious. I rubbed healing herbs on his feet, the only part of his body that was free of tubes. We demanded quiet in his room. We didn't permit anyone to turn on the television or radio. We brought in a little stereo and played healing music nonstop.

We also refused to let the doctors and nurses discuss his condition in front of him. We were quite adamant about it. From their viewpoint, his body simply wasn't functioning, nor would it ever function. It's human nature to be influenced by other people's perceptions, especially by those we regard as experts, and even more so in situations as grave as this. If the doctors' fixed expectations of Josef's damaged brain were the only reality offered to him, then I'm sure my son would have become vegetative. We didn't want his spirit to get too attached to these perceptions and obstruct the vast healing potential that's available to all of us. Josef told us that he was coming back with the full force of his spirit and vitality intact, and we believed him. We knew, in fact, that his remarkable healing journey would only make him a much stronger person, one more fully engaged with spirit.

While he was in a coma, my communications with him existed outside of the body, in a spiritual realm. Although he was unconscious, when a medical procedure needed to be performed, I would explain his options to him so that he could make choices about his healing. Each time his body would improve so that the intervention was no longer necessary. For instance, his doctors wanted to install a breathing tube in his throat because they were concerned about infection if he remained in the coma for a long time. I told Josef he had two choices: He could wake up out of the coma or have the tracheotomy. The next day he showed the first signs of regaining consciousness. To this day, Josef and I are uncannily in tune with each other. When he was mountain climbing in Nepal a few years ago, I would sense when he was going to call, so I'd make sure I was home and waiting by the phone. Every time, he would call.

Every step of the way was slow and arduous. When Josef

regained consciousness, he was like an infant. He had no motor control; he couldn't talk, walk, or even hold his head up. He was a flop of a body slumped in a wheelchair. Despite the nurses' fears that he would choke, I began feeding him while he was still receiving intravenous nutrition. I know my son. He loves to eat. And an amazing thing happened. We discovered that he was ravenous! Using an eyedropper, I fed him herbal teas and fresh carrot juice. It took him hours to drink even a small amount of juice, but his hunger further awakened him and brought him back to his body.

Once he could swallow, I fed him small spoonful by small spoonful of carrot juice, miso soup, yogurt, and oatmeal that I made each day and brought to the hospital. While this food was more vital than chemical nutrients passed into his veins, it also fed his will to live. For all the breakthroughs and scientific leaps Western medicine has achieved, hospitals are still woefully in the dark when it comes to nourishing patients. How can we expect sick people to heal if they're fed lifeless foods—refined sugars, highly refined flour products, processed foods, and devitalized produce—when those same foods cause physical disturbances in healthy people?

I believe that all my prior training and experience with nourishment, healing, and spiritual growth was a preparation for this moment. This was my initiation. I learned from my son how people can heal—body, heart, mind, and spirit. When Josef was comatose, it was clear that machines could maintain his body for a long period of time, for a lifetime if necessary. But the body is merely an empty husk without the animating force of spirit. In many spiritual traditions, spirit is closely associated with breath. In fact, the word *spirit* comes from the Latin word *spiritus*, which means "breath." For Josef to embody spirit, he literally needed to make his body strong enough to breathe and function on his own.

Witnessing Josef's recovery, I learned how people respond to healing if they are provided optimum nourishment at all levels. Today Josef is a physically robust, intelligent, adventurous, and gifted college student. He's the kind of person who jumps out of bed at the crack of dawn and swims a mile or two. He loves to help people, and has a passion for other cultures, traveling, and cooking. How do I explain what even the specialists regard as his miraculous recovery? Certainly his medical care is one factor. Another is Josef's intense will to heal and become a fully functional, integrated person again. This will made it possible for me to work with him those first weeks, months, and years. Don't misunderstand me. A couple of glasses of carrot juice didn't heal him. Ultimately, Josef healed himself. I simply provided the nourishment to support his body's natural ability to rebalance itself—vital, potent foods, unconditional love, and the absolute knowing that he could become whole and strong.

If Josef could recover from a nearly fatal head trauma and a month-long coma, it shows us the body's incredible power for healing. Thankfully, most of us will never have to endure what my son went through. At all times, no matter the state of our physical condition, our bodies are always seeking balance. The body wants wholeness. It's designed to make micro-adjustments to maintain equilibrium, its natural sense of ease. The more ease we feel in our bodies, the more we can feel, listen to, and express our spirits.

ACCEPT THE CHALLENGE WITH A GRATEFUL HEART

Spirit is vast as the ocean. Just as the seas gave birth to the first life forms on earth and shaped continents, so, too, our spirits have the potential to grow and transform our lives. Saying yes to our spirit is one of the most daring things that we can do in life, if not the most courageous. Every time your true self is challenged, you will always be supported. The right person or the right circumstances will suddenly appear. The right job. The right book. The right words uttered by a coworker or stranger standing next to you on the subway. That's because the natural impulse of spirit is to become manifest. Of course bad things happen, and they do happen to good people. As Josef's story shows, none of us is free from crisis or hardship.

When you're aligned with your spirit, your whole life opens up. What this means is that you feel deeply connected to a source of wisdom that exists within you, that guides you and helps you develop your unique gifts and talents. Ultimately, the spirit's work is without attachment to ego and is always for the benefit of all. It's done for the sake of the work rather than your own sake. Certainly in the process you also benefit, but the motivation comes from the desire to be a vehicle for inspiration, change, and creativity. If we allow the body to be what it is born to be—vital, harmonious, and flexible—then it's easier to do the spirit's work.

Our challenge is to live life to the fullest, even when life gets hard. Buried among the pain and hardship of life's difficulties— divorce, death, illness, financial challenges—are the jewels for incalculable personal and spiritual growth. I couldn't possibly have known that I was going to be presented with a life and death situation while driving a car pool one afternoon. If I did, would I have done anything differently? If I hadn't been 100 percent committed to my son's healing, would he have been vegetative? Would I have learned the inner lessons of healing and transformation that I teach today? Josef's accident has profoundly shaped everyone in our family; in our own ways, we each understand that life is a gift not to be wasted.

There's an illusion that spiritual life looks a certain way. A spiritual life is when everything happens magically and we have it together at all times, right? This is an illusion. Those of us living non-monastic lives with families, professions, relationships, and financial responsibilities are being asked to integrate our spiritual work into our daily life. Nourishment is one way to help us embody spirit. Of course embracing your spirit can be scary, just as deciding to get married can be frightening because you're making a long-term commitment. Until this commitment is in place, however, spirit can't fully emerge in our lives. Making the commitment to our spiritual growth is an acknowledgment that we are not alone in the world, that we are not the sole driving force of our lives. To become vehicles of spirit we must be willing to receive the words of our soul. At first we nourish ourselves for our own growth, but ultimately our deep purpose is for the healing of the world.

EVERYDAY HOLINESS

I was driving in my car recently when I switched on the radio just in time to catch the tail end of an interview with Bishop Desmond Tutu on a National Public Radio talk show. A caller had just asked Bishop Tutu his opinion of the condition of humanity's goodness. This program aired about six months after the attacks on the World Trade Center in New York. If you look at humanity's goodness from that lens alone, the picture is fairly bleak. Bishop Tutu said something that deeply resonated with me. "I actually think the world is looking out for holiness," he said. "We should be striving to have more people who are holy, people who are prayerful, people who are compassionate, who allow the compassion of God to work through them."

To be holy, prayerful, compassionate, and a vehicle to manifest divine works seems like a tall order. Certainly it's not for the faint of heart. For centuries, the clergy fulfilled this role in many societies. While the world's religious traditions are one place to look for expressions of holiness, I understand Bishop Tutu's remarks to mean that we are ready for the sacred to become more integrated into our daily lives. In fact, I would put it in more urgent terms. People today are desperate for meaning and fulfillment. We hunger for rich inner lives and long to feel connected to ourselves, to one another, and to the divine. In Bishop Tutu's words, "we are looking out for holiness" in others as well as in ourselves.

Humanity in its fullest expression is a spiritual consciousness. The quality of our lives, the well-being of the world's societies, and the very health of our planet depend on our ability to regularly touch our souls and fulfill the acts of spirit. In the West, we place a lot of value on developing the mind. Now it's time to develop the spirit, to drop below the surface and look more deeply into our lives. How do we nurture this inner stirring? We're lucky; we don't have to lead monastic lives or become saints to gain spiritual fulfillment. We can choose from so many paths today. Prayer life. Meditation. Yoga. Self-awareness practices. Spending time in nature. Performing acts of service. If your spirit is nurtured by any one of them, then commit firmly to that path because it is pure nourishment for you.

You've heard it said that the body is a temple. Well, it's true. Our culture has become so appearance-obsessed, it would like us to believe that our bodies are nothing more than a clothing size. But I tell you that the body is sacred. Our spirits don't exist free from our bodies, at least not while we're alive on this earth. Our spirits require a home, and that home is the physical body. Your body is nothing short of the holy dwelling place for your spirit. One way to grow our spirit is by fully, lovingly, and reverentially nourishing our bodies. In this way ordinary people, people like you and me, can embody spirit in our everyday lives.

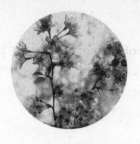

PART TWO

NOURISHMENT AS
DAILY PRACTICE

4

VITAL ESSENCE FOODS

Eating is a sacrament. The grace we say clears our hearts and guides the children and welcomes the guest, all at the same time. We look at eggs, apples, and stew. They are evidence of plentitude, excess, a great reproductive exuberance. Millions of grains of grass seed that will become rice or flour, millions of codfish fry that will never, and must never, grow to maturity. Innumerable little seeds are sacrifices to the foodchain. A parsnip in the ground is a marvel of living chemistry, making sugars and flavors from earth, air, water. And if we do eat meat it is the life, the bounce, the swish, of a great alert being with keen ears and lovely eyes with foursquare feet and a huge beating heart that we eat, let us not deceive ourselves.

—GARY SNYDER, *from* The Practice of
the Wild

Dinner in my home begins with everyone in the kitchen. Since the time my children were very young, I've always engaged every family member in the preparation of our meals. From opening a can to washing potatoes, stirring a pot, taking out the compost, and setting the table, everyone is part of the meal. Sitting down at the table has always been a special time for our family. No matter what's going on in our lives, dinner is an opportunity to come together. We light a candle and hold hands. Either someone offers a blessing over the food, or we silently make our own individual blessings. And then we eat.

Tofu. Fish. Rice. Fresh salad greens harvested from my garden with edible flowers. Different vegetable dishes made from leeks, cauliflower, carrots, green beans, and potatoes from an organic family-run farm about ten miles from our home. Our experiences in the kitchen are ones of wholeness that begin and end with the vital foods we feed ourselves. Because we've all interacted with the food—picking it from the garden, going to the farm stand, purchasing it at the store, cooking it in the kitchen—there's a real joy and appreciation for the beautiful meal before us.

Food comes directly from the source of all life. Certainly people are integral to the process of cultivating and producing food, but like all forms of life, plants and animals are gifts from the divine. Because our food comes from the source of life, it gives us an opportunity to connect to the divine each and every time we place something in our mouths. In this way, food not only supports our physical sustenance, it can also nourish our spiritual development. To support our spiritual development, along with our physical and emotional well-being, we need to feed ourselves foods that are as close to the source as possible. These are *vital essence foods*: foods that are available in their appropriate season and have undergone little to no processing or chemical treatment. In this way, eating vital essence foods is more than a set of food guidelines, it's a way to recover our natural instincts about how to nourish ourselves.

In addition to a food's basic nutrients, when we feed ourselves, we also ingest the *essence* of a food—how it was grown, harvested, stored, transported, cooked, and assembled. Even the attitude of the person cooking your food affects its quality. Because foods like organic produce, whole grains, and freshly caught fish retain their original integrity, their essence remains *vital*. Their life force is vibrant, feeding us the direct energy of the elements—sun, rain, wind, and earth. Since most of us don't grow our own food or have the opportunity to spend time in nature, consuming vital essence foods is a profound way to regularly connect to the earth.

When a food is stripped of its natural qualities, it loses this vital essence. The food may contain the same nutritional components, but its life force has been compromised. How do you feel after you've eaten a potato that you've baked in your oven compared to a bag of potato chips? The essential ingredient is the same: potato. But once the potato has been chopped, salted, fried, produced in mass quantity, and packaged in a factory by someone you don't know it has lost most of its life force. On the other hand, the fresh potato that you've baked in your oven still contains its potato-ness: The potato looks like itself, has a wonderful warm, earthy smell, and each mouthful fills you with a sense of hardiness and being rooted in the earth. You may also feel the satisfaction of having prepared it for yourself, as simple as turning on an oven and baking a potato may be. Lifeless foods make us dull in body and spirit. Vital foods energize us, awakening our body and spirit to a sense of passion, creativity, and meaning in life.

Feeding ourselves vital essence foods doesn't mean that we never eat potato chips or that we live solely on raw salads. We do, however, need to make sure that we feed ourselves vital essence foods on a regular basis. For example, if you're purchasing a week's supply of yogurt, consider buying the organic brand. In this day and age, it simply isn't realistic to expect that every food or meal is seasonal or organic. So what can you do? You can become aware that you have a choice about what you put into your body. Each time you select produce in the grocery store, a drink from the vending machine, or a meal from a restaurant menu, you're making the decision for that food or beverage to be *your* food and to become part of *your body*. For this very intimate reason, it's important to become an informed consumer.

Before purchasing a product, do something as simple as reading the label. Even if you can pronounce all of the ingredients, you may be shocked by the fine print. For example, Tropicana apple juice advertises to be 100 percent juice. But if you read the label, you'll discover that a twelve-ounce Tropicana bottle is made of apple concentrate from ten countries spanning four continents: Germany, Austria, Italy, Hungary, Argentina, Chile, Brazil, Turkey, China, and the United States. When you consider that each continent has different climates, growing seasons, and quality controls, let alone the amount of fuel necessary to transport the apples across the globe, you may think twice before buying this juice. Learn more about agricultural and food production practices so you can make informed decisions about those that you are willing to support—with your dollars and your body.

THE WISDOM OF THE SEASONS

Would you feed yourself a pineapple in the cold of winter? Baked yams on a ninety-degree day in summer? Did you know that a domestic apple purchased in March most likely was picked the previous September, when it also was waxed and chemically treated to sustain cold storage so that you could eat it six months after it came off the tree?

Only forty years ago, Americans ate mostly in harmony with the seasons. Local, seasonal vegetables and fruits were essentially the only fresh produce you could obtain—from your own backyard gardens or local markets. Imported produce was a luxury. With the advent of cold storage methods and modern supermarkets, "fresh"

VITAL ESSENCE FOODS

Feed yourself local, seasonal produce so that you establish a connection to the earth's rhythms and feed yourself in harmony with the seasons. When possible, purchase organic produce, grains, and free-range or hormone- and antibiotic-free animal products. Establish a relationship with the source of your food by knowing the geographical area where it was grown and who prepared or cooked it before it ends up on your kitchen table.

Vital Essence Foods Include:

- Organic seasonal vegetables and fruit
- Whole grains
- Seeds and nuts
- Beans and legumes
- Tofu and soy products, non-GMO
- Fish, caught in the wild
- Free-range chicken and eggs
- Hormone- and antibiotic-free meat and dairy products
- High-quality olive oil, canola oil, flax oil, and sesame oil
- Purified drinking water

produce from around the world became available all year long in virtually every corner of the United States. That's why even during blizzard conditions in Buffalo, you can brave your way to the supermarket and purchase honeydew melons (from Mexico), oranges (from Florida or California), and avocados (from California or the Dominican Republic).

In the supermarket, seasons don't exist; or, rather, everything is in season all the time. The availability and abundance of produce is now so commonplace, we expect to walk into a market and buy anything we want whenever we want—from tropical fruits to berries and mahimahi fish from Hawaii. This isn't to say that modern-day supermarkets don't have their advantages. But the price of convenience, abundance, and variety is that we've become out of touch with the seasons. I always ask my clients to tell me what they think is growing in a particular season. About 95 percent of them tell me they have no idea. And they aren't alone. Unless you're a gardener, farmer, or otherwise attuned to nature, seasonality means what's on the supermarket shelves—which is nearly everything all the time! The problem is that when we're disconnected from the fundamental earth wisdom of what is growing and how that food affects us, it becomes more difficult to ascertain what we should choose to feed ourselves today. It's like being in a windowless room for a long time; you don't know if it's day or night, if it's time to sleep or to be awake.

When you feed yourself according to the seasons, you are connected to nature's life cycles—the earth, climate, and the growing seasons. Plants have an inherent wisdom in that they will only grow when the conditions are appropriate, providing the perfect sustenance to the people who live in that climate. The basic principle is that foods grown in a hot or warm climate usually have a cooling effect on the body, which helps keep the body regulated in warm weather. Likewise, warm foods that grow in cooler climates have a warming effect on the body, which is needed to maintain warmth in cold weather. For example, melons, corn, cucumbers, and tomatoes grow in the hot summer months. The high water content makes these foods quick to digest and have a cooling effect on our bodies. In the cooler months, starchy vegetables grow, such as potatoes, yellow turnips, cauliflower, and winter squash. These vegetables contain more carbohydrates, so they are digested more slowly to create longer lasting heat in the system.

Let's take a closer look at this relationship between the seasons, food, and our bodies. Have you ever noticed that you tend to gain weight during the cold winter months? That's because we're usually less physically active during the colder, darker months and instinctively feed ourselves foods that are higher in fat and starch to insulate our bodies from the cold. Starting with Thanksgiving, people tend to eat more animal products and refined carbohydrates such as baked goods. When the weather is warmer, our bodies don't require much insulation. The first spring vegetables that grow are bitter greens. Vegetables such as chives, sorrel, spinach, dandelion greens, kale, watercress, green onions, and arugula all have cleansing properties. The bitter taste of these greens isn't just a flavor for our taste buds. The bitter taste stimulates increased liver functioning, which helps the body break down and eliminate any excess fat stored during the winter so that our bodies will be refreshed and lighter in preparation for the warmer months ahead.

What happens when you feed yourself out of season? Let's say you order a plate of sliced melons for breakfast at a restaurant in Chicago in January. We've been programmed to believe that fruit is always a healthy choice, but before taking a bite, consider the conditions this particular fruit grows in. Melons, like cantaloupe, watermelon, and honeydew, grow in a very hot climate. It's fine if you order this fruit in August, when it could grow in Illinois, but in January melons most likely are being imported from a tropical country like Mexico. For approximately ninety days, these melons have been growing in intense heat, gathering the essence of the tropics to fuel the people in Mexico with the exact sustenance they need for their climatic conditions.

Melons have an especially cooling effect on the system, which is necessary in a hot climate. If we transport that melon to Chicago in January, where it's freezing cold and people are wearing long underwear and bundling in heavy jackets to maintain heat, this cooling food will create an immediate imbalance in the body. One piece of melon may not make a difference. Your body may even be able to digest a few slices periodically during the colder months. But regularly feeding yourself foods that are out of season can lead to a number of imbalances, such as lethargy, lowered immunity, excess weight retention, and other digestive disturbances. In this way, a vital food harvested in January for the locals in Mexico actually has a detrimental effect for those in Chicago.

If you don't know what grows in your area, take it upon yourself to find out. Ask your local grocer or contact your state's department of agriculture. To give you an idea of when vegetables and fruit are growing in a particular region, the following chart lists some of the vegetables and fruits that grow where I live in New England.

Choosing seasonal produce means that we're mostly consuming what's grown locally. Of course, it isn't possible to get fresh, local produce year round in every part of the country. In colder climates where the growing season is shorter, we have to make the best choices we can. In the past, our ancestors would have supplemented their winter fishing and hunting efforts by storing produce from the fall harvest in cold cellars or curing vegetables and fruits by salting, drying, smoking, canning, jamming, and pickling them.

I'm not advocating that we emulate our ancestors entirely and forgo shopping in the supermarket. However, we can learn from their example by mostly choosing foods in the wintertime that would have grown during the previous season—such as turnips and other root vegetables, winter squash, leafy green vegetables, apples, and pears. This doesn't mean that you never eat a grapefruit from Florida if you live in New Jersey. As with other aspects of feeding yourself, you simply need to pay attention and make sure to choose a variety of foods that are appropriate to the season, climate, and location where you live.

SAMPLE NEW ENGLAND HARVEST SCHEDULE: FRUIT

	JUN	JUL	AUG	SEP	OCT
Strawberries	●				
Blueberries		●	●		
Nectarines			●		
Peaches			●		
Melons			●	●	
Grapes			●	●	
Raspberries				●	
Apples				●	●
Pears				●	●

SAMPLE NEW ENGLAND HARVEST SCHEDULE: VEGETABLES

	JUN	JUL	AUG	SEP	OCT
Salad greens	●	●	●	●	●
Cooking greens	●	●	●	●	●
Lettuces	●	●	●	●	●
Radishes	●	●	●	●	●
Herbs	●	●	●	●	
Peas		●			
Cucumbers		●	●	●	
Summer squash		●	●	●	
Beets		●	●	●	●

	JUN	JUL	AUG	SEP	OCT
Cabbages		☻		☻	
Green beans		☻	☻	☻	
Onions		☻	☻	☻	☻
Broccoli		☻	☻	☻	☻
Celery			☻	☻	
Corn			☻	☻	
Eggplants			☻	☻	
Carrots			☻	☻	☻
Peppers			☻	☻	☻
Potatoes			☻	☻	☻
Leeks				☻	☻
Cauliflower				☻	☻
Pumpkins				☻	☻
Tomatoes				☻	☻
Turnips				☻	☻
Winter squash				☻	☻
Parsnips					☻

THE WISDOM OF ORGANIC FOODS

When you think about it, feeding ourselves is a very intimate experience. We take external matter—lightly sautéed chard with olive oil or fresh plump raspberries—inside our bodies, and it becomes us. Because food so profoundly affects our well-being, we need to pay very close attention to the conditions under which it is cultivated, as well as to the unwanted hidden ingredients that we may inadvertently be consuming, namely chemicals and hormones.

Pesticides. Genetically modified foods. Bovine growth hormones in dairy and meat products. The corn on the cob, pat of butter, grilled chicken, and spinach salad on your plate may contain a lot more than you've bargained for. Sadly, most of the food grown today for mass market has been chemically treated or altered for the primary purpose of producing higher yields at less cost and greater profit for the manufacturers. The only way to keep up with production for the market at such great quantities is to use chemical intervention. For the animals and earth to create more, we are sacrificing natural rhythms, the integrity of the life that's cultivated for food, and the vibration of the foods that we feed ourselves.

When you produce more than the earth can naturally yield, you create excess, and that excess is toxic: chemicals in the soil; pesticides in fruits, vegetables, and products derived from contaminated produce; hormones and antibiotics in dairy and meat products; and far-reaching problems with our earth, air, water supplies, and ecosystems that only now are being understood. When we feed ourselves foods produced against the grain of natural rhythms, we perpetuate that pattern of excess within our own bodies. On the one hand, we are consuming toxic chemicals, which have been linked with various forms of cancer, learning disabilities, reproductive problems, immune disorders, and other health problems. On a more subtle level, our bodies and spirits also are affected by the stressful conditions under which the earth and animals are forced to overproduce.

When food is grown to create more, we need to consider the magnitude of the intervention used to increase production, from the chemicals that are used to how the earth and animals are treated. The food yielded from synthetic intervention is produced with a certain amount of stress to the soil and animals. The continual spraying of pesticides, chemical fertilizers, and monoculture—the cultivation of a single crop—depletes the soil. To produce more, animals also have less—chickens are debeaked and crowded into small cages; cattle, pigs, and lambs are kept in tiny pens with no fresh air or the ability to exercise. (Eric Schlosser's *Fast Food Nation* is an excellent study of the inhumane practices of today's meat industry.)

Let's stop a moment and consider how stress affects us. Today, stress is the number one cause of many current physical ailments—from gastrointestinal distress to difficulties with conception, migraines, and heart disease. You know how it feels to be under pressure to produce or perform under multiple deadlines, with too much to do in too little time. What happens? Maybe you can tolerate this fast pace for a while, but eventually you will burn out. Burning out is just another way of your body, mind, spirit, your whole self, saying, "Stop, take a break." Unfortunately, the animals and the soil don't have that freedom; they are continually driven to produce without any regard or sensitivity for their living nature. So, you see, a cycle emerges. As humanity continues to experience more and more stress, we continue to stress our natural resources, and we then consume the products of that stress, which leads to more stress for people.

I know this creates a rather bleak picture, but we do have

choices. We can break the cycle. How? By taking responsibility for our nourishment and becoming educated about how our food is cultivated so we can make informed decisions about the foods that we ingest and the type of production we support economically. We know what it means to be smart consumers. We'll spend a lot of time shopping for cars, computers, electronic equipment, cameras, sporting gear. When my son Micah wants to purchase stereo equipment, he'll devote hours to researching the latest technology, reading magazines, searching the Internet for the highest quality at the lowest price. If we can be such savvy consumers when it comes to purchasing electronic equipment or household appliances, then isn't it possible to be as informed about the products that we *literally* consume?

Our earth doesn't have to be poisoned to yield food for us; nor does the basic, daily act of feeding ourselves mean that we have to consume toxic chemicals. Even though the use of chemicals has become pervasive in large-scale farming, it is possible to feed ourselves foods that are cultivated with reverence for the earth, respect for animals, and regard for human health. This is the wisdom of organic foods. How are "organic" foods different from other kinds of food when it all basically comes from the earth? Organic foods are those grown closest to natural rhythms as possible—cultivated in fertile soil and without synthetic or genetic intervention.

How does the apple you picked at a nearby organic farm look compared with the hundreds of apples in the supermarket? The supermarket apple will be large, shiny, and the skin is a consistent color without blemishes. This apple looks exactly like all the other apples in the bin. It's a perfect-looking apple, worthy to tempt Adam. But don't be fooled. In nature, "perfect" unblemished fruit is rare. The organic apple, on the other hand, is smaller, has a duller sheen, the skin is a subtle blend of several colors, and no two apples on the tree look exactly alike. While this apple may not look as pretty, it's a much closer relative to the tree in Eden.

Organically grown food and products made with organic ingredients are now available in virtually every part of the country. It's even possible to order organic foods through the Internet. Guidelines also have been established to regulate the criteria for what constitutes "organic" vegetables and fruits. One way of ascertaining if your produce or food item is organic is by looking for the label "Organically grown and processed in accordance with the California Organic Food Act of 1990."

Because organic farms are smaller and more labor intensive than commercial factory farms, organic foods do tend to be more expensive. For those of us living on budgets, organic foods may seem a luxury. One way to reduce your costs and simultaneously support organic farming is by purchasing a "share" in community supported agriculture (CSA), where you prepurchase that season's produce from a local organic farm. Or you could choose to buy organic products for the produce that's known to contain the most pesticide residues. According to the Environmental Working Group, a Washington-based not-for-profit environmental research organization, apples, peaches, pears, strawberries, and green beans typically have the highest levels of pesticides.

But don't let the decision to purchase organic produce be an obstacle to feeding yourself more vegetables and fruits. In this day and age, I find that we can't be purists about everything. For many people, simply expanding their daily amount and variety of vegetables will be a significant step toward improved nourishment without worrying about buying everything organic. As long as you are an aware consumer, you can make the informed choices that are appropriate for you.

At the same time, however, I can't emphasize enough the importance of organic poultry, beef, and dairy products. The hamburger on your plate and the seemingly pure white milk in your glass don't tell you the whole story. The only way to raise livestock at the high volumes and speed at which they are fattened for market is to give them cheap feed and to inject them with antibiotics and growth hormones, such as synthetic estrogen. Dairy cows are also given bovine growth hormones (BGH) to create more milk than bovinely possible, and at the expense of udder infections, for which they are treated with antibiotics. All of which is passed along to you, the consumer.

For these reasons, if you choose to feed yourself meat and dairy products, it is particularly important that you purchase organic. Organic meat comes from animals that are fed organic feed, given space to roam, and are not injected with growth hormones and antibiotics. Following the principle that we should feed ourselves the most natural foods, so, too, meat should be derived from animals that have been permitted to live as natural a life as possible. Ideally, this means that the animal has been given adequate living space, the ability to exercise, fresh air, and good feed. It would stand to reason that the better cared for and healthier the animal, the healthier the food derived from that animal will be.

Does all of this mean you have to feel fearful about everything you put in your mouth, toss out the food in your refrigerator, and purchase all organic foods tomorrow? Absolutely not. Nourishing yourself simply means taking responsibility for the food you put into your body. Read labels. Learn more about how and where your food was produced. What was its life cycle before it arrived in your kitchen? Taking a more active role in your own well-being also leads to greater responsibility for your participation in the food chain: The choices you make about your food play a role in the quality of our soil, air, water, farm workers, animals, and the future availability of vital food.

TAKING RESPONSIBILITY
FOR YOUR FOOD

Think about what you ate yesterday. Out of everything you ate or drank, how much do you know about where your food came from or whose hands actually participated in preparing it for you? If growing or raising your own food is the most direct link to your food source, then a fast-food hamburger, Coke, and fries is the furthest removed. The ingredients that go into making the fast-food meal come from various countries, farms, ranches, slaughterhouses, chemical laboratories, and processing facilities before arriving for assembly at the fast-food chain.

When we obtain the majority of our meals from delis, cafés, restaurants, and fast-food chains, or assemble meals from boxes, cans, and frozen packages at home, we are the least connected to our food's source. Being disengaged from the direct process of feeding ourselves means that we relinquish control of our food source to other people. Sometimes the person providing our food is a well-intentioned chef who uses quality ingredients, but most of the time it's not a "person" at all but a host of anonymous people, assembly lines, and questionable ingredients, including the attitude of the individuals handling the food.

The less control you have of your food source, the less responsibility you take for your nourishment. We see this in the animal world all the time. Animals in the wild hunt or graze only when they are hungry, whereas domesticated animals, or animals in captivity, tend to overeat and eat out of boredom. Except for ani-

mals in confinement, every animal, including humans, can instinc-
tually regulate how much to eat and when to feed. The more control we have of our food source, the more we reconnect to our
natural instincts that know when we're hungry, the appropriate
foods for that hunger, and how much we need to be truly satisfied.

For his entire life, my client Antoine never cooked for himself.
Living in the city, he ate out, ordered in, or had food prepared by his
wife or personal chef. Motivated by health concerns, one year he
decided to do a cleanse while vacationing and away from his normal
routine. He quickly discovered that most restaurants don't serve
cleanse foods and that he would have to take care of his own food
preparation. For the first time, this sixty-five-year-old man, who
didn't even know how to scramble eggs, had to cook. I gave him
some basic kitchen guidance and he was motivated to try it. When
he came home from his vacation, he called me. "I've had a break-
through," he said excitedly. "I realized that only I know what I really
need. If I want to feel healthy and vital, then I can't just expect others to provide for me. I have to provide for myself." For Antoine, taking responsibility for feeding himself made him feel better physically.
It also empowered him to know he could rely on himself.

There are a few ways we can reclaim control of our food
source. While not everyone can grow their own food or has access
to a local farm or farmer's market, we are all capable of food shopping and preparing at least some meals for ourselves. I think everybody senses there's something inherently nourishing about a
home-cooked meal. When my children come home, they are always
grateful to be fed vital food that has come right off the stove or out
of the oven. Indeed, prepared foods, like Campbell's Simply Home
soups and Ragú tomato sauce, capitalize on this connection when
they boast that their product is home-cooked style, or "the next best

thing to Mama," as Ragú's advertising claims. These products play off the idea that a home-cooked meal is a nourishing one. And it's true. If you were sick with the flu, which would you choose to feed yourself: soup from a can, soup from the deli, or soup that your friend made for you from scratch that very day? Home-cooked meals made with fresh ingredients not only taste better, they also *feel* better because we know that somebody cares enough to prepare the meal, including if that somebody is ourselves.

When you regularly shop and prepare your own food, you become a source for knowing what, when, and how much you need to feed yourself. Taking responsibility for feeding yourself also furthers your discipline and dedication to nourish and care for yourself in every other way. Today, the most common obstacle that prevents people from cooking is time. At least that's the chief complaint I hear over and over again.

Actually, it's an illusion that it takes more time to prepare food for ourselves than to dine out or purchase ready-to-eat products. If the kitchen is the least familiar room of your house, then, yes, initially it will take some time to learn how to shop, organize, and cook. Cooking doesn't mean that you suddenly have to produce culinary masterpieces in your kitchen every day. I advocate keeping it simple most of the time, unless of course you're inspired to be more creative and elaborate. For instance, yesterday was a very busy day and I didn't have a lot of time to prepare dinner, so I made a relatively simple meal: lentil soup, roasted potatoes, and sautéed greens, which we had with leftover salad greens from lunch. This satisfying, tasty, and nourishing meal took about half an hour to prepare. You can find the recipe for that lentil soup in the back of the book, as well as for many other simple and delicious meals that take under an hour to prepare and cook.

5

DAILY PRACTICE

Work. Keep digging your well.
Don't think about getting off from work.
Water is there somewhere.

Submit to a daily practice.
Your loyalty to that
is a ring on the door.

Keep knocking, and the joy inside
will eventually open a window
and look out to see who's there.

—RUMI, *from "The Sunrise Ruby"*

WHAT DO I NEED TO FEED MYSELF?

It's dinnertime. You're standing in your kitchen, opening and closing every cabinet. You open the refrigerator for the third time, hoping for a miracle. But no such luck. It's exactly the same assortment of Tupperware containers, old condiments, cartons, and packages that were there a moment ago. Nothing looks satisfying. So you just stand there in the middle of the kitchen, hungry and having no idea what to feed yourself. At one time or another, most of us have been completely bewildered in our own kitchens, or in a restaurant, or in the market. It's amazing just how much of a dilemma this is. What do we need to feed ourselves right now?

Deep down, we all know how we *should* feed ourselves. Sometimes I'll ask my clients to list all the foods they think they should have as well as the ones they're currently consuming. Most of the time these lists look very different. What do people think they should feed themselves? Just what you'd expect: more fresh vegetables, fruit, lean proteins, and whole grains, and less sugar and refined foods. If we already have this awareness, then why is there such a gap between how we know we should take care of ourselves and how we actually live?

For as long as I can remember, the food pyramid has instructed us to eat a variety of fruits and vegetables every day. This advice appears so straightforward, so simple, yet it doesn't seem to penetrate our collective understanding of how to feed ourselves. While statistical studies may indicate that Americans are eating the USDA's recommended servings of three to five vegetables a day, a closer look reveals shocking information about how the government classifies vegetables and what people actually are feeding themselves. "And although the number of vegetable servings appears close to recommendations, half the servings come from just three foods: iceberg lettuce, potatoes (frozen, fresh, and those used for chips and fried), and canned tomatoes. When fried potatoes are excluded from the count, vegetable servings fall below three per day," reports Marion Nestle in her groundbreaking book *Food Politics: How the Food Industry Influences Nutrition and Health.*

With more Americans overweight and obesity at epidemic proportions, it's become clear that physical health isn't enough of an impetus for people to make changes. I don't know anybody who wants to be regarded as just a mechanical, physical body. So, too, we need to shift our awareness of health from the physical to the total person—body, heart, mind, and spirit. Only then can we make the connection that the food we ingest directly feeds all parts of ourselves, thereby profoundly influencing the quality of our lives.

In this chapter we will explore ways for nourishing yourself to stay calm, balanced, energetic, and connected to your spiritual life force. Instead of being bewildered in front of the open refrigerator, you can learn how to feed yourself exactly what you need in each moment to nourish yourself as a spiritual being. Not what your mind thinks you should have. Not what your sweet tooth craves. Not what your loneliness longs for. Not what's easiest to grab. But what your spirit needs to grow and thrive in this body.

Getting in touch with this inner awareness sounds like a pretty good proposition, right? But how do you go about making it real? Every artist, composer, architect, schoolteacher, scientist, and gardener has a set of tools specific to their field. So does nourishment. In this chapter I present you with a set of practical tools for learning how to feed yourself. These simple strategies have been distilled from years of hands-on work with clients and research into various healing systems. Essentially, I have incorporated Japanese and Chinese medicine and philosophy, naturopathic nutrition, and herbal medicine into accessible daily practices that can be adopted into people's busy lives.

If you feel compelled to experiment with this way of feeding yourself, please resist the urge to undertake everything all at once, starting this Monday. Needless to say, developing self-awareness, shifting your relationship to food, and changing twenty-five or fifty years of feeding behavior takes time. Even though I've been doing this for a long time, I'm always learning something new about my body and the foods that best support my growth. Be patient. The most important thing is that you are willing—open to experiment, explore, play, willing even to get it all wrong and to try again the next day.

TIPS FOR DAILY PRACTICE

1. Give your body a rest from digestion so it can have a chance to repair and rejuvenate itself. A twelve-hour rest from digestion is ideal, so try not to eat after 7:00 P.M. or 8:00 P.M.

2. Simplify and ease digestion through food combining (see page 90).

3. Ask your body what it needs in this moment. Take the cues from your body—not what it craves, not what your mind wants, but what you genuinely need for strong energy and mental clarity.

4. Fuel up instead of fill up. Use the fuel test to notice how you feel one to two hours after a meal. Is your energy still strong? Your thoughts clear? Heart open? If so, then you know that food is good fuel for you.

5. Increase the amount of land vegetables and sea vegetables to keep your body and spirit feeling light and vibrant.

6. Free yourself from the salt and sugar pendulum by expanding the tastes you eat every day: sweet, salty, bitter, sour, and spicy.

7. Don't just feed your taste buds; let food nourish all of your senses. The more engaged you are with the smells, textures, colors, even with the sounds of your food, the more deeply food will satisfy you and the less likely you will be to overindulge.

8. Prepare ahead by keeping healthful snacks in your purse, briefcase, backpack, desk, or with you while traveling.

LIGHTENING THE LOAD: EASY DIGESTION

In my lifelong exploration of nourishment, I've discovered that the key to keeping our bodies and spirits light is through easy digestion. When you eat a meal, let's say chicken with pasta and cream sauce, you may not think much more about the food after it's been chewed and swallowed. But chewing and swallowing are just the beginning of your body's digestive process. For several hours after you've finished your chicken and pasta, the body will continue to digest that meal, creating the digestive juices to break down food-stuffs, assimilating nutrients, and eventually eliminating any excess material that cannot be used for fuel. By eating complicated food combinations, processed foods, or simply too much food, we essentially force our bodies to work overtime to try to digest everything that we've put into it.

Most of us think about digestion only when it's *in*diges-tion—bloating, gas, heartburn, constipation, and all the other unpleasant symptoms that quickly direct our attention to our digestive tract. A whole pharmaceutical industry has evolved for the sole purpose of treating indigestion. If you're prone to heart-burn, simply chew a tablet and you can continue to feed yourself the same foods that don't agree with your system. While I don't advocate anyone remain needlessly in pain, these products allow us to treat the symptoms and continue perpetuating the same behav-iors that caused the problem in the first place. Indigestion is usually the body's way of saying, "Whoa. I can't make sense out of these foods," or, "The system is on overload."

The fundamental purpose of food is to provide us energy— energy for walking, talking, thinking, being creative, running in the park with our children, living our lives. This same energy is also used for digesting food. The more energy that's required for diges-tion, the less energy we have for living. We ordinarily expend a great deal of energy digesting foods that are difficult for our system— these include processed meats and foods that are fried, refined, loaded with sugar, salt, and chemicals. When people consume less of these foods and more vital essence foods (see chapter 4) that are easier to digest, they're always amazed by the increase in their vitality. Instead of all the energy they normally would have needed to just digest their food, that energy is freed up for other areas of their lives. My client Charles remarked that since he has increased vital foods in his diet, he has a lot more energy. "It's energy for the most clear and creative thinking I've ever done. I look at all the food that's available in the supermarket and out on the street, and I think there's no way I would trade how clear and uncomplicated I feel for anything."

All together, the length of the digestive tract—from mouth to esophagus, stomach, small intestine, large intestine (colon), and anus—is twenty-five to thirty feet. We've all learned basic biology in school, but I find that most people forget just how extensive the digestive system is. When I show clients an illustration of the digestive tract, I can almost see the light above their head switch on. Seeing the illustration drives home the understanding that what goes into the mouth stays in the body a long time.

The American diet of rich meals, refined and processed foods, and overindulgence—coupled with a sedentary lifestyle—basically forces the factory of our digestive system to work around the clock. What would happen to any machine that's operating at full tilt twenty-four hours a day, seven days a week? Eventually, that machine will break down. The same is true for the body. For the body to repair cellular structure and maintain health, it needs a chance to rest from the demanding job of digestion. Ideally, we should give ourselves a twelve-hour break from digestion each day. This means that if you feed yourself breakfast at 8:00 A.M., for example, then you shouldn't eat any more food after 8:00 P.M.

When a person eats a diet comprised regularly of processed foods, refined flour products, meat, dairy, and sugar, a sticky plaque can form and adhere to the intestinal walls. This excess matter creates obstacles that block the assimilation of nutrients and prevents proper elimination. If elimination doesn't happen regularly (one to two times a day) waste matter can remain in the system, which can create great toxicity. When we overburden our digestive tract in this way, we feel uncomfortable and lethargic; the flow of life energy is blocked. In my practice, gastrointestinal ailments are by far my clients' chief complaints.

When we feel lethargic, we think the only way to increase energy is by doing what we've always done—turn to sugar and caffeine for stimulation. Today you can even obtain instant energy from countless bars, power drinks, powders, and vitamin packets. Only a decade ago, these items were specifically intended for athletes and available mostly at specialty vitamin stores. Now my local drugstore carries a whole display of these power bars right next to the candy section. There's nothing wrong with using these items occasionally, but such highly processed products can never replace the benefit of feeding yourself primarily vital essence foods.

So how do we keep life energy flowing? The answer is by making it easier for the body to break down food, absorb nutrients, and expel waste matter. We can achieve optimum digestion by feeding ourselves mostly vital essence foods and foods in the combinations that are easiest to digest. Instead of expending so much energy on digestion, the body then has more energy for the elimination of waste matter and the rejuvenation of cellular structure. Increased physical energy means more vitality and attention for all areas of your life. Essentially, the lighter we feed ourselves, the lighter we feel.

FOOD COMBINING

If you think of the stomach as a food processor that purees food into a molecular soup that gets poured through the rest of our digestive tract, then what we eat at one meal doesn't matter. It all gets mashed up together anyway. What difference does it make? Experience with hundreds of clients, in fact, has shown me that there is a difference. Time and time again I have seen that feeding ourselves the appropriate combinations helps improve digestion, increase energy, regulate elimination, release emotional blockages, and free up energy for deeper self-inquiry and reflection. Food combining has come in and out of public attention in recent years, popularized by *Fit for Life* and other diet books. With food combining, digestion is easier and more efficient because you eat foods that require the same gastric juices and have compatible digestion times.

While food combining can get quite complex, I find that a few key guidelines are all that's necessary to understand this sound way of feeding yourself for easy digestion. The food combining model presented here isn't necessarily the strictest version you will find. To make this way of feeding ourselves practical for a diverse range of people, I've developed an approach that's more flexible than other schools of thought on the subject. For example, strict food combining advocates separating starchy vegetables from proteins, whereas experience shows me that people have longer-term success with food combining when they can have a starchy vegetable with their fish or chicken dinner. After you try food combining for a while, you will have a clear sense of the combinations that do and do not serve you.

FOOD COMBINATIONS

- Fruit eaten alone
- Vegetables with vegetables
- Grains with vegetables
- Protein with vegetables

FRUIT (digestion time: 20–60 minutes)

Fruits are the easiest and fastest foods to digest, and for that reason should always be eaten separately from proteins, grains, and vegetables. Due to their acidity and sugar content, fruits are further classified into acid, subacid, sweet, and melons, and have their own set of guidelines for combinations.

VEGETABLES (digestion time: 30 minutes to 2 hours, depending on starch content)

Vegetables include non-starchy, low-starchy, and starchy vegetables. All vegetables can be combined with one another, as well as with protein. It's best to combine only non-starchy and low-starchy vegetables with grains.

GRAINS (digestion time: 2–3 hours)

Grains can be eaten alone or combined with non-starchy and low-starchy vegetables. Grains should not be combined with protein, and it's best to avoid combining them with starchy vegetables as well. It's best to have only one grain at a meal, so decide if you really want that hunk of bread or if it's worth waiting for the delicious brown rice and mushroom dish (see recipe page 245).

FOOD COMBINING FOR EASY DIGESTION

Non-starchy and Low-starchy Vegetables

Arugula
Asparagus
Bok choy, pak choy, tat soy
Broccoli
Brussels sprouts
Cabbages (red, green, napa, savoy, Chinese)
Cauliflower
Celery
Chard
Collard greens
Corn (fresh)
Cucumbers
Dandelion greens
Eggplant
Green beans
Kale
Leeks
Lettuces
Mesclun greens
Mizuna greens
Mustard greens
Onions
Peas
Peppers
Radishes (red, black, daikon)
Scallions
Sea vegetables (arame, dulse, hiziki, nori, wakame)
Shiitake mushrooms
Spinach
Sprouts
Summer squashes
Tomatoes
Watercress
White turnips

Starchy Vegetables

Beets
Burdock
Carrots
Jerusalem artichokes
Parsnips
Potatoes
Rutabaga (yellow turnip)
Sweet potatoes
Winter squashes
Yams

Proteins and Fats

Avocado
Beans
Eggs
Fish
Milk and dairy products
Nuts
Olives
Poultry
Red meat
Seeds
Tofu and soy products

Grains

Amaranth
Buckwheat
Millet
Oats
Quinoa
Rice
Spelt
Wheat and flour products

PROTEIN AND FATS (digestion time: 2–4 hours)

Protein can be eaten alone or combined with non-starchy, low-starchy, and starchy vegetables. It's best to have only one protein at a meal.

From hamburgers and hot dogs to wraps, subs, hot pastrami, steak and cheese, peanut butter and jelly, bagels and cream cheese, BLTs, veggie burgers, and egg McMuffins, sandwiches are easy, portable, and fast. They're at the heart of American eating. But have you ever felt sleepy after eating a sandwich and wondered why? If you have a sandwich at noon every day, chances are you'll start itching for a cup of coffee or a sweet around three o'clock, and that's not just because you're restless and need an excuse to get up from your desk! One of the reasons you may feel tired and unfocused is because grains and proteins are one of the most complicated combinations to digest. When combined with our sedentary lifestyle, the daily sandwich simply provides poor sustenance for most adults today.

Simplifying your digestion through food combining is one of the easiest ways to enter the daily practice of transformational nourishment. The basic rule of thumb is that the simpler the meal, the easier digestion will be. The word *digestion* comes from the Latin for *separate* or *arrange*. In fact, this is exactly what happens within your digestive tract: In simple terms, your body separates nutrients (in the form of molecules) from food and arranges them (through assimilation) to provide energy and revitalization for all of your body's internal organs. With food combining, you actively assist digestion by separating and prearranging your food through certain combinations before the food even lands in your stomach.

FRUIT COMBINING FOR EASY DIGESTION

Because of the acidity and sugar concentration of different fruits, certain fruit combinations are easier to digest. Acid fruits combine well with sub-acid fruits; subacid combine well with sweet; but the acid and sweet fruits are not a good combination. Due to their particularly high water content, melons are the fastest to digest and therefore should be eaten alone.

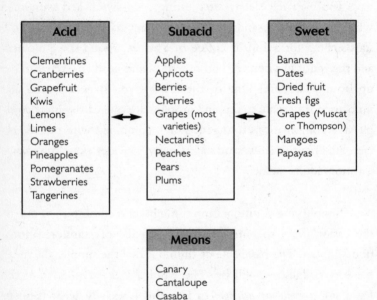

Acid	Subacid	Sweet
Clementines	Apples	Bananas
Cranberries	Apricots	Dates
Grapefruit	Berries	Dried fruit
Kiwis	Cherries	Fresh figs
Lemons	Grapes (most	Grapes (Muscat
Limes	varieties)	or Thompson)
Oranges	Nectarines	Mangoes
Pineapples	Peaches	Papayas
Pomegranates	Pears	
Strawberries	Plums	
Tangerines		

Melons
Canary
Cantaloupe
Casaba
Christmas
Honeydew
Musk
Persian
Watermelon

FEEDING WHOLENESS

THE FUEL TEST

With the abundance and variety of food available to us all the time, how do we begin to make sense of what to feed ourselves? I personally know many people who would be quite relieved if they had far fewer food options to choose from each day. I've discovered that the "fuel test" is one easy way to begin discovering how to feed ourselves. The purpose of the fuel test is to discern your most potent food sources so you can purposefully fuel up and not just fill up.

The main guideline for ascertaining if a food fuels you well is the answer to the question: How do I feel one to two hours later? If your energy is still strong, if you feel vibrant, focused, and emotionally balanced, then you know that particular food is good fuel for you. If you feel lethargic, irritable, unable to focus, and crave more of that same food, then you know that that food depletes you. Pay attention to how particular foods like sugar, caffeine, carbohydrates, protein, vegetables, fats, and fruit affect you so that you can begin to discern the foods that serve you or sap you of your life force.

THE NOURISHING MAGIC OF VEGETABLES

Remember your parents telling you to eat your vegetables when you were a child? They were telling you a great truth. Of all the food families, fresh vegetables are among the easiest foods to digest. When I say vegetables, however, I'm not talking about soggy broccoli or canned peas. Nor am I referring to the piece of wilted lettuce and the few onion and tomato slices on your hamburger or sandwich. I'm talking about real, vital, hardy vegetables that inspire life, vigor, and a sense of well-being that you can feel radiate from your stomach to the crown of your head, fingertips, and toes. From roots to leafy greens and vegetables that grow in the sea, vegetables are one of the most diverse food families on the planet.

In terms of basic biochemistry, vegetables are one of the easiest types of food to break down, assimilate, and ultimately use as fuel, because their structure converts easily into glucose, which our bodies use for energy. Because we digest fresh vegetables so efficiently, our bodies generally don't store them as excess matter. Of course, we can't and shouldn't rely solely on vegetables as our only source of energy; we also need slower-burning types of energy from fats, proteins, and other carbohydrates to function throughout the day. All I'm recommending is that fresh vegetables be a significantly larger part of our daily consumption.

When my Japanese friends visit me in Boston, they're always overwhelmed when we go out to eat. They're shocked by the portions. The typical American meal consists of a big piece of protein, a medium serving of grain or other starch, and a small side dish of vegetables. I say, break the mold. Turn the American diet on its head and simply reverse the proportions. In his most recent book, *Eat, Drink, and Be Healthy,* Walter Willett of the Harvard School of Public Health has replaced the out-of-date U.S.D.A. Food Guide Pyramid with a new Healthy Eating Pyramid based on extensive research at Harvard. What does this sane new pyramid emphasize? You guessed it, an abundance of vegetables. So make vegetables the centerpiece of your meal, with smaller amounts of protein and grain, and your body will thank you.

When I go to the supermarket, I can't help but peer into people's shopping carts to see what they're buying, something that used to embarrass my daughter quite a bit. No matter where I am in the country, the standard lineup of vegetables going into the cart is tomatoes, cucumbers, lettuce, broccoli, frozen peas, frozen corn, and frozen green beans. I understand this pattern. It's easy to fall into the habit of purchasing foods and products that you're familiar with. You run out of that one item and it automatically goes onto your shopping list, so that you're forever replacing just the same few items.

If you feel that vegetables are lackluster and a chore, it's probably time to widen your vegetable horizons. Have you ever tried a purple potato (sweet and starchy); daikon radish (fresh and pungent); dandelion greens (yes, they're edible!); or even a classic, earthy rutabaga (at one time, the staple root vegetable in many parts of the world)? I personally love to try new vegetables, particularly when I'm traveling. It's like taking a new way home instead of going the same old route. The next time you go to the supermarket or farmers' market, go on a food adventure and leave your grocery list at home. Spend time in the produce aisle investigating all the vegetables that are on display. Look at the various dark leafy greens, varieties of potatoes and starchy vegetables, turnips, lettuces, leeks, sprouts, winter and summer squashes, Asian cabbages, and radishes. If you're drawn to a vegetable that you've never tasted before, ask the grocer about its taste and preparation methods, or find a recipe in a cookbook.

SEA VEGETABLES: EDIBLE SUNKEN TREASURES

As the potency of our earth continues to be depleted by overgrowing and chemical pesticides, we need to look elsewhere to find naturally occurring sources of vitamins and minerals. Fortunately, we don't have to look too far. Our oceans are teeming with life—vegetable life, that is.

The next time you're in a Japanese restaurant, consider this before you munch on your sushi roll. Sea vegetables (seaweed) are excellent sources of calcium, iodine, iron, phosphorous, potassium, and other trace minerals, as well as many vitamins. Sea vegetables help regulate the thyroid and adrenal glands, and also are fantastic for promoting the health of your skin, hair, and nails. Why are sea vegetables such a miracle food? As Paul Pitchford points out in his book *Healing with Whole Foods*, human blood contains all 100 or so minerals and trace elements that exist in the ocean. He writes, "Seaweeds contain these in the most assimilable form because their minerals and elements are integrated into living plant tissue. In fact, as a group they contain the greatest amount and broadest range of minerals of any organism, and hence make superb mineral-rich foods." These foods are so potent, they've even been documented to remove radioactive and toxic metal wastes from the body.

If you think of seaweed as an odd delicacy found only on the menus of Asian restaurants, think again. Did you know that the Iroquois Indians of North America used dried seaweed instead of salt? Or that seaweed has been used in Europe and South America for centuries? In fact, anywhere the oceans produce these mineral-rich gems, people have harvested them.

Today, most sea vegetables can be purchased dry in health food stores or Asian markets. Sea vegetables vary in taste and consistency. Because they are so rich in minerals, even a small amount will benefit you. I encourage you to test the waters, so to speak, and experiment with delicious and nutritious sea vegetables like wakame, dulse, hiziki, arame, and nori, which you may already recognize from the sushi bar. I know that seaweed can be somewhat intimidating to the novice sea vegetable eater, so I've included easy and tasty recipes in the back of the book to help you take the plunge.

THE FIVE TASTES: THE SPICE OF LIFE

> If people pay attention to the five flavors and blend them well their bones will remain straight, their muscles will remain tender and young, breath and blood will circulate freely, the pores will be in fine texture, and consequently breath and bones will be filled with the essence of life.
>
> —*THE YELLOW EMPEROR'S CLASSIC OF INTERNAL MEDICINE* (NEI CHING)

Our very first taste is sweet: the taste of mother's milk or baby formula, juice, fruit juices, cookies. We naturally identify this as a good taste, so good that many of us develop an insatiable sweet tooth later in life. In this country, the two tastes that predominate are sweet and salty. People tend to fall into two camps: "sweet" people or "salty" people, though occasionally someone is equally compelled by both. Think about the foods and drinks you're drawn to in the course of the day. How many fall into the category of sweet or salty?

Traditional Chinese medicine identifies five categories of taste and recommends a balance of these flavors each day for optimum health. These tastes are sweet, salty, bitter, sour, and spicy/pungent. The flavors don't need to be consumed in exact proportion; the important thing is that you have at least some small amount of bitter, sour, and spicy foods each day to balance the larger quantities of sweet and salty flavors.

The five tastes teach us that there's a whole world of taste outside of the familiar salt and sugar characters that we all know and love so well. Let's take a closer look at what they are.

Sweet. This is one of the most obvious tastes. Ice cream, cake, cookies, candy, baked goods, fruit, sodas. But the sweet taste also pertains to carrots, potatoes, rice, corn, tomatoes, red peppers, and peas. Sweet is the most readily available taste of all the five flavors. And it's the one we turn to most often for comfort. For some people, sweet is the only taste they ever develop, and it becomes their downfall. Sweet cravings seem to have a life of their own. Unless we get serious about reining them in, they will continue to live quite greedily within your body. If you find yourself plagued with sweet cravings, try sour- or bitter-flavored foods and drinks for a quick antidote. Because of their cleansing properties, foods such as lemons and dark green bitter vegetables like kale, watercress, and arugula cut the sweet cravings.

Salty. Table salt is just one example of the salty flavor. Salty foods also include miso (fermented soy paste), sea vegetables, pickled vegetables, and some cheeses. The salty flavor is the polar opposite of sweet. For this reason these two tastes frequently go together. French fries and a Coke. Beer and pretzels. For people who consume a lot of sweets, the only way they know how to balance their bodies is with salt. Salt is an important mineral, yet in this country, salt is dramatically overused. Like sugar, salt is a flavor enhancer that sneaks into almost all processed and packaged food, let alone the liberal use of the salt shaker in your own home or restaurant.

Bitter. The bitter taste exists in many green vegetables, particularly the cool-weather greens such as arugula, asparagus, collard greens, broccoli rabe, dandelion greens, kale, scallions, mint, basil, and snow peas. Bitter foods aid in digestion and are cleansing to the system. As such, they provide an excellent balance to the extremes of salt and sugar excess.

Sour. The sour taste can be found in citrus fruits like lemons, limes, and grapefruits, as well as sour pickles, sauerkraut, Granny Smith apples, and certain green vegetables like parsley and sorrel. At the taste of sour foods, most of us pucker up. Sour foods aid digestion by creating an acidic medium in the stomach that helps break down fats and protein. The sour taste also acts as an astringent and helps cut down on excessive food cravings. If you're a person who tends to crave dessert after a meal, consider drinking a glass of hot or room-temperature lemon water to ease the need for sweets.

Spicy/Pungent. Cayenne, chili, jalapeño peppers, cinnamon, fennel, ginger, garlic, radishes, turnips, and onions. Are you beginning to sweat a little? This flavor is highly stimulating to our system: It aids circulation and turns up the heat of our digestive fire. Spicy and pungent foods open our pores and make us sweat, which is one way to draw out toxins, making spicy foods particularly beneficial to people who don't get a lot of exercise. For those who are sensitive to spicy foods, you can still play with this taste by using the more mild flavors of cinnamon, fennel, sweet onions, and turnips.

FEEDING YOUR SENSES

Now that we've explored a range of tastes, let's consider all the ways that we can connect to food in addition to taste. Obviously, taste is our most immediate and palpable understanding of food, but we have four other sense faculties with which to perceive and interact with our world. The more we can open all of our senses to food, the more deeply nourished we will feel.

Smell. Fresh-brewed coffee. Homemade tomato sauce simmering on the stove all day. Onions sautéing in a pan. Fresh-baked cookies. A lemon. Our sense of taste is inextricably linked to our sense of smell. When I was in college, I cooked in a natural foods restaurant. At that time I was actively experimenting with various cleanses, so I wasn't eating any of the foods the restaurant served. Because I couldn't taste what I prepared, I had to rely solely on my sense of smell. To this day I usually don't taste my food while I'm cooking. I let the smells inform me how to adjust and fine-tune the ingredients.

Sight. When we look at a beautiful landscape or exquisite painting, we say it's a feast for the eyes. For centuries painters have depicted the natural beauty of fruits and vegetables. When we eat in gourmet and avant-garde restaurants, we take great pleasure in the chef's culinary artistry. Yet if we feed ourselves quick meals, it's usually at the sacrifice of our sense of sight. It's important for people to engage regularly with beauty, and food is one way we can literally consume it. Texture. Shape. Color. Nature has provided us an incredibly wide color palette. Even within the same color, there are myriad variations. Notice all the gradations of the color red, for instance, from strawberry red to the red of a Fuji apple, pepper, radish, cherry tomato, raspberry, and plum. The next time you feed yourself, open your sense of sight and allow yourself to truly feast.

Touch. When children are young, they actively explore the world first through taste and then touch. We, too, can engage in the world of food through touch, not only with our hands, but also with our mouths. Touch has to do with engaging in the process of preparing and feeding yourself food: holding, weighing, selecting your vegetables and fruits; chopping, grating, kneading, stirring. Touch allows us to develop a relationship to food, which is another way to actively participate in our nourishment.

Within our mouths, we can explore a whole range of textures—creamy, crunchy, smooth, lumpy, tough, chewy, substantial, dry, greasy—and understand how each of those textures makes us feel. Because we have to exercise our jaw, crunchy foods tend to activate our will and determination. On the other hand, smooth, creamy foods give us the feeling of comfort and the sense memory of being taken care of when we were young children. One day my client Louise announced that she'd had an epiphany while eating a bowl of borscht the night before. "Now I understand texture and not just taste," she told me. "If I want something nourishing, I can have something creamy like applesauce or goat cheese. I can be satisfied by texture and not just the quantity of food."

Sound. The sound of food? Yes, it's even possible to develop awareness of our food's sounds. Of course, this sense has more to do with the process of preparing a meal than it does the actual sound of a bunch of spinach. In the modern, convenient kitchen, the sounds of meal preparation are all electronic: the microwave beeping, can opener whirring, blender, food processor, coffeemaker. The less mechanized our food production, the more subtle and pleasing the sound. The next time you cook, really pay attention to all the sounds involved: the knife hitting the cutting board as you chop vegetables; soup bubbling on the stove; fish sizzling in the oven; oil sputtering in the pan; the sound of water running from the faucet.

THE SUGAR AND WHEAT DOLDRUMS

Sugar and wheat are siblings in the same family—the family of foods that don't support us. These two ingredients creep quietly and stealthily into many processed foods. Sugar is the particularly cunning sibling. All processed wheat products contain sugar—bread, crackers, cereals, muffins, bagels. Even salty wheat products like pretzels contain sugar.

Sugar isn't just the white granules you stir into your coffee: Sugar also means corn syrup, high-fructose syrup, fruit juice, orange juice, ketchup and tomato sauce, soft drinks, and on and on. Sugar has become so pervasive in the American diet today that serious warnings continue to be issued about the health dangers of its overconsumption. According to the United States Department of Agriculture (USDA), people consuming 2,000 calories a day should have only about 10 teaspoons of added sugar. But USDA surveys show that the average American consumes about twenty teaspoons of sugar per day. To put this figure into perspective, consider that soft drinks alone contain nine teaspoons of added sugar per twelve-ounce serving.

Children are the most vulnerable to this sugar epidemic, and soft drinks are one of its most insidious forms. "A 12-ounce can contains about 1.5 ounces of sugar and 160 calories, but so little nutritional value that the Center for Science in the Public Interest rightfully refers to soft drinks as 'liquid candy,'" writes Marion Nestle, chair of the Department of Nutrition and Food Studies at New York University, in her book *Food Politics*. "From 1985 to 1997, school districts decreased the amounts of milk they bought by nearly 30% and increased their purchases of carbonated sodas by an impressive 1,100%."

Children aren't the only ones drowning in sugary soft drinks. According to the Center for Science in the Public Interest, "In 2001, Americans spent over $61 billion on soft drinks. The industry produced 15 billion gallons of soft drinks, twice as much as in 1974. That is equivalent to 587 12-ounce servings per year or 1.6 12-ounce cans per day for every man, woman, and child. Soda pop is Americans' single biggest source of refined sugar, providing the average person with one-third of their sugar."

Of course you would expect soft drinks to contain a lot of sugar, but like my clients you may be surprised to learn of another concentrated form of sugar you just may be drinking every morning at breakfast. One of the first things I tell all of my clients is to stop drinking orange juice. My clients are shocked when they hear this. Their mouths fall open. Everyone thinks orange juice is good for you. It seems so healthy and pure. But did you know that orange juice contains the same sugar content as some sugar-sweetened sodas? A twelve-ounce serving of orange juice made from frozen concentrate contains forty grams of sugar, the same quantity as Coke and Pepsi, according to research cited in Nestle's *Food Politics*. Even orange juice that's not from concentrate contains over thirty grams of sugar per twelve-ounce serving. If you want to drink orange juice, squeeze your own, but drink the juice of only one orange. You may be surprised by how little juice one orange actually yields. While it's true that orange juice is a source of vitamin C, there are many other sources of vitamin C, including grapefruits, lemons, green vegetables, berries, and sweet peppers.

If you start your day with sugar—a bagel, muffin, bowl of cereal, orange juice—then you will end your day with sugar. Because sugar is so addictive, it sets you up in the morning, and it sets you up for failure. Sugar wreaks havoc on our bodies by suppressing the immune system. If we're consuming a lot of sugar in the form of processed foods and soft drinks, then we're less likely to have the fresh vegetables and proteins that supply our body with a variety of nutrients. Not only does sugar compromise our physical health, it also creates serious imbalances in our emotional and spiritual alignment. You can never win with sugar. It sucks out our life force. When we're addicted to sugar, we're constantly driven to feed our habit, to get the next pleasure fix. This incessant pleasure-seeking clouds our thoughts and takes our awareness away from the present moment.

Wheat has a similarly addictive effect. We think of bread products as low fat, and therefore allow ourselves far too many highly refined carbohydrates in the course of the day. Before they started working with me, some of my clients had to have three to four bagels a day. Most people in this country simply have an excess of refined flour in their bodies, which causes addictions and allergies. When people eliminate wheat, they experience fewer cravings. It's that simple. Ask yourself how you would feel about not having any bread or flour products tomorrow. Or how would you feel about not drinking soda or other soft drinks. Be honest with yourself. If your first thought is, "No way, I can't do that!" then that's a clear indication of an addiction to wheat and/or sugar.

Before we can access our sense of spirit, we have to be honest and willing to make changes. This doesn't mean that if you decide not to eat wheat tomorrow you will never be able to have wheat again. When I work with people to break their dependence on sugar and wheat, they will try to get very crafty and bargain with me. "Does this mean I can have whole wheat pasta?" No. If you know deep down that you've become ensnared by the wheat and/or sugar trap, then the only way out is through steady discipline. If you wish to explore a daily discipline to help you learn more about your own particular patterns, see chapter 6 on cleansing.

PUTTING IT INTO PRACTICE: SUGGESTIONS FOR GENTLE FOOD OPTIONS

Substitute Food Options

- *Bread:* Rice cakes; spelt bread; sprouted essene bread

- *Coffee:* Organic black tea; roasted green tea; licorice tea; ginger tea

- *Corn chips:* Organic blue or yellow corn chips; potato chips baked or fried in olive oil; root vegetable chips

- *Fruit yogurt:* Plain or vanilla organic yogurt; goat yogurt; sheep yogurt

- *Ice cream:* Frozen yogurt and ice cream that doesn't contain bovine growth hormones (BGH); natural sorbet; soy or rice frozen desserts

- *Milk:* Rice milk; almond milk; oat milk; soy milk

- *Orange juice:* The juice of one pink grapefruit*; the juice of one orange

- *Pasta:* Rice noodles; spelt pasta; Japanese soba or udon noodles

- *Peanut butter:* Almond butter; hazelnut butter; sesame butter

- *Soft drinks and fruit juice:* Sparkling water with lemon or lime; spring water; herbal iced tea

- *Sugar:* Maple syrup; rice syrup; honey; date sugar; raw, unprocessed sugar

*Please be aware that grapefruit juice should not be consumed with certain prescription medications. Ask your physician or pharmacist about possible interactions with your prescription.

Simple Comfort Foods

- Applesauce (see recipe page 287)
- Baked apples or pears (see recipe page 285)
- Fresh, seasonal berries with a dollop of plain or vanilla yogurt
- High-quality herbal, green, and organic black tea with soy milk
- Hot soup
- Organic dried fruit (nectarines; pears; apples; apricots)
- Protein smoothie (see recipe page 282)
- Rice cakes with almond butter
- Rice cakes with apple butter
- Roasted root vegetables with oil and salt (see recipe page 240)
- Warm almond or soy milk with cinnamon

Essential Pick-me-ups

- Baby carrots
- High-quality herbal, green, and organic black tea
- High-quality, non-tropical tree nuts—almonds; walnuts; hazelnuts
- Organic dried fruit (nectarines; pears; apples; apricots)
- Organic yogurt
- Pumpkin seeds; sunflower seeds
- Sea vegetables—wakame and nori
- Spring water with lemon

Staples for the Office

- Apple butter and almond butter
- Bottled water
- Canned fish—tuna; salmon; sardines
- High-quality, non-tropical tree nuts—almonds; walnuts; hazelnuts
- Hummus, black bean, and other bean dips

- Miso paste or single-serving cups of miso soup
- Organic yogurt
- Raw, precut vegetables
- Rice cakes
- Sea vegetables—wakame and nori
- Single-serving protein drinks
- Tea bags and your own mug

6

THE CLEANSE:
A RETREAT INTO YOURSELF

*Refining energy into spirit means keeping the clear and
removing the polluted.*

—THE TAOIST CLASSICS, *volume 3*

Before my clients embark on a cleanse, I tell them, "What
you're about to undertake is a retreat into yourself." When you're
on a retreat, you normally go someplace where you don't have to
worry about your regular life. No work. No deadlines. No phone.
No e-mail. Just time to be still with yourself. To do a cleanse, you
don't have to go to a lavish retreat center or a remote mountain-
top—although that does sound pretty good. To cleanse, you don't
have to go anywhere except inside yourself. Of course, it's more
challenging to create a retreat-like environment while you have to
keep up with the rest of your life. But if undergoing a cleanse
while maintaining your daily responsibilities presents certain challenges, it also has its rewards.

Most of us live very full lives. My clients are doctors, teachers, lawyers, artists, students, mothers, fathers, people taking care of
their elderly parents. The cleanse has to work *within* their daily
lives. To do a cleanse, you have to make a certain time commitment
as you learn how to prepare food, shop, and feed yourself in this
new way. But the cleanse's structure is supportive. You won't col-

lapse under its demands. Chances are you will feel more energized and vital. And, most important, you will get an immediate understanding of how to integrate nourishment into your everyday life.

The foods we normally eat—processed and refined foods, fried foods, caffeine, sugar, white flour products, red meat, and dairy—put a lot of strain on our internal organs. The body has to work overtime to digest, assimilate, and eliminate these complicated foodstuffs. To make matters worse, we place our bodies under even more stress by regularly overeating and not getting enough physical activity.

The twin goals of the cleanse are to eliminate excesses from the body (toxins, impacted plaque in the intestines, and bacteria) and increase the body's natural ability to renew itself through the rejuvenation of cellular growth. Cleansing is like giving your body an annual tune-up. Once or twice a year we need to give the body a rest from our regular eating patterns so that it can eliminate old cellular material, reenergize, and rebuild itself. In this way, we give our bodies a well-deserved and much-needed break.

As the body releases toxins and begins to renew itself, people usually get the desire to cleanse what is "toxic" or excess from all parts of their lives. This takes shape differently for different people. Some people are motivated to break addictive food patterns. Others have ended unfulfilling relationships or had sudden realizations about their careers. Women in particular learn they can make time every day to take care of themselves, rather than allowing other people's demands and schedules to run their lives.

I've helped hundreds of people cleanse, and over the years I noticed a pattern in what people said about their experiences. Many people told me that they obtained a level of clarity and self-control they never felt before. Bonnie used to be in the pattern of constantly eating foods that she didn't really want. She would catch herself in the act of eating a candy bar, knowing it wasn't going to make her feel good, but she couldn't stop. After cleansing, she said, "Now I'm in control. It's not that I never have sugar, but I have a choice. I'm the one deciding what to eat."

One of the most important benefits people gain from the cleanse is learning that it's possible to make positive changes. I would say it's more than possible; it's almost guaranteed. At the end of each cleanse, I ask my clients to describe the benefits they derived from following this discipline. Physical changes range from improved digestion, regular bowel movements, and weight loss to clear skin, better sleep, and increased energy.

But the physical changes are just the beginning. After three weeks of cleansing, my clients also report that they feel more confident and proud of themselves than they have in a long time; know how to take better care of themselves; have clear thoughts and better attention; feel calm and in control of their lives; and generally have a more positive outlook on life. These changes are nothing short of remarkable because they occur within only three short weeks. After finishing his first cleanse, Pablo said, "You can't call it the cleanse, it's the transformation!" Of course, like anything, for the seeds of change to grow, they must take root in our daily lives. More than anything, the cleanse offers you a taste of what life can be like when you nourish yourself with this much awareness and love not just once a year but all the time.

I have been teaching food and consciousness since 1975, and it has become clear to me that there isn't one single way to cleanse. For millennia, the self-healing practice of cleansing has been a regular part of the world's religious traditions and healing systems. I was first drawn to the idea of cleansing when I was seventeen. My interests were spiritual in nature as much as they were physical. It was 1967 and like others of my generation I had become interested in purifying my body as a way to help me grow spiritually. When I began to investigate physical purification practices, the most prevalent ones written about were strict fasts, where one consumed only water or juice.

From 1967 to 1974, I experimented with numerous fasts. In 1974, I became a fruitarian and fed myself only fruit for seven months. I was adamant about this way of eating, and refrained from having even one tiny sunflower seed. After seven months of eating only fruit, my future husband and I decided to do a fast together, and we consumed only water and freshly made fruit juice for forty days. The concentration of fruit sugar over such a long period of time caused my face to break out in severe acne. Soon after that fast I began to eat a macrobiotic diet, which contains a lot of salt. Because my body was so out of balance from the fruit, I blew up like a balloon. I was suddenly enormous. My body was completely out of balance, and the sudden introduction of salt in my system caused me to retain fluids. It was quite dramatic.

From these extreme experiences, I learned how *not* to cleanse. I kept to the fruitarian diet and forty-day fast strictly out of willpower. During that entire period, my body couldn't retain heat, and I was freezing cold all the time. But I wasn't listening to my body. I was intent on following those diets no matter what. Because I was seeking spiritual attainment outside of the physical, I believed I could transcend the body and its needs. Fortunately, because I was so young, I could withstand the extremes I forced my body to endure. I eventually realized that the spirit and body don't exist separately, and that we can't afford to ignore the body.

I would never recommend that anyone cleanse the way I did when I was younger. The valuable lesson I learned in 1974 is that we need to work *with* the body to create spiritual and emotional balance, and to do that we have to learn how to respond to our bodies' needs. On this earth, we exist in bodies. If we don't use this vehicle properly, the whole system—our bodies, minds, hearts, and spirits—will be out of balance.

Over the past twenty-five years, through research and work with clients, I have developed a sensible and gentle food-based cleanse that people can incorporate into their daily lives. Numerous cleanses and detox diets exist. The cleanse I offer provides a structure for people to connect to their own truth of what they need to feed their bodies, emotions, and spirits. This model evolved over years of experience and has proven to be extremely potent for people. One of the reasons it is so effective is because it is moderate and balanced; people get a taste of how good they can feel when they feed themselves simple, whole foods in the appropriate combinations.

I want to emphasize that like anything having to do with the body, cleanses are individual. Your body is dynamic, literally changing moment by moment. What's important is that you respond to your body and how it feels right now. Bemoaning that a cleanse he had done for many years no longer supported him, a client said to me, "I followed the exact principles of that cleanse for many years. Initially I lost weight, but over the years when I followed the same cleanse, I didn't lose any more weight."

There was nothing wrong with my client's cleanse. Over the years his body simply changed, as do all of ours. I've been cleansing for over thirty years, and each cleanse is a different experience. What nourished me well when I was eighteen didn't necessarily serve me at twenty-eight or forty-eight. So, too, your body may respond differently to the cleanse from one year to the next. Once you understand how to listen to your body, you will know how to modify the cleanse each year to support the person you are today, not the person you were two years ago. I invite you to follow the cleanse guidelines outlined here, but please remember that they are only guidelines. Your body's own wisdom should always be your ultimate authority.

The cleanse may not be appropriate for everyone. If you are pregnant, have a serious illness, or are under a doctor's care, you should not undertake a cleanse. If you have any concerns about cleansing, please consult your health professional. If you're taking any medications or vitamins, you should maintain your normal regimen while cleansing.

HOW THE CLEANSE WORKS

I learned that so much of my energy was needed just to digest all the food I had been eating, which left me feeling tired, foggy headed, and out of it. Once I simplified my digestion and cleared out the junk, most of that energy was freed up for me to use elsewhere. I have never felt so clear headed, creative, joyful, grounded, peaceful—I could go on and on! And I can't ever imagine diverting the energy that produces these good feelings back to my digestion. That is why I will continue eating this way for the rest of my life.

—CHLOË

I'm always surprised when people automatically assume the cleanse is a fast. Nothing could be further from the truth. In fact, fresh, whole foods are the star players of this twenty-one-day cleanse.

Just as the wrong foods can bog us down, the right ones can help us naturally and gently cleanse and rejuvenate the entire gastro-intestinal system. Instead of expending so much effort on diges-tion, the cleanse gives your body more energy for the elimination of waste matter and the rejuvenation of cellular structures.

OVERVIEW OF THE PHASES OF THE CLEANSE

Preparation: **1–2 Weeks**

A preparation period alerts your body of your intention to cleanse and mitigates any potential reactions caused by the sudden release of toxins into your bloodstream. One to two weeks before your cleanse, significantly reduce or eliminate your intake of toxin-forming foods, including processed foods, refined flour products, caffeine, alcohol, sugar, red meat, and milk. If you are hooked on coffee, gradually decrease your caffeine consumption by lessening the amount of coffee, or try switching to a caffeinated black tea and then to a green tea.

Phase 1: Vegetables & Fruit **1 Week** *(or 2–6 days)*

By consuming only simple, easily digested foods, this first phase of the cleanse gives your body a chance to release any stored excesses—toxins, impacted plaque in the intestines, and bacteria.

Phase 2: Grains, Seeds & Nuts **1 Week** *(or 2–6 days)*

Small amounts of whole grains and seeds are added to your daily consumption of vegetables and fruit. These building foods provide just enough protein and complex carbohydrates to help you perse-vere with the cleanse while maintaining the responsibilities of your daily life.

Phase 3: Protein **1 Week** *(or 2–6 days)*

With the addition of protein, you gently transition to a more inclu-sive way of feeding yourself. Many people maintain this third phase for much longer than a week, and some even use it as the model for feeding themselves on a regular basis.

See page 118 for a list of cleanse foods and page 187 for cleanse recipes.

The focus of the first part of the cleanse is on the release of toxins, impacted plaque in the intestines, and bacteria that's trapped in the system. If it's difficult for you to imagine intestinal plaque, then just think about your teeth. Even if you brush your teeth twice a day, excess bacteria and mucus can cause plaque to build up. Just as your smile can benefit from regular dental cleanings, so, too, your intestines need to be cleansed to maintain health. Of course, we can't brush our intestines, but we can help them release old matter by consuming an abundance of chlorophyll- and mineral-rich vegetables. During the second and third phases of the cleanse we'll gradually add back the more complex grains and proteins that help rebuild cellular structures.

We know from food combining that optimal digestion, assimilation, and elimination occurs when we simplify the foods that we eat together in one meal. Organized in three phases, the cleanse, too, follows this model of food combining (see chapter 5 for an indepth explanation of food combining). Each phase of the cleanse typically lasts one week, so the total length of the cleanse is twenty-one days, plus a one- to two-week preparation period. If a twenty-one-day cleanse is more of a commitment than you can make in your life, you may modify the length to suit your particular needs. Some individuals shorten the cleanse to seven, ten, or fourteen days; for example, a ten day cleanse could be organized as phase one (three days), phase two (two days), and phase three (five days).

CLEANSE FOODS

The following chart offers you a range of cleanse food choices. For delicious and easy cleanse recipes, see the recipe section at the end of the book.

VEGETABLES

NON-STARCHY AND LOW-STARCHY VEGETABLES

Arugula

Asparagus

Bok choy

Broccoli

Brussels sprouts

Cabbages (red, green, napa, savoy, Chinese)

Cauliflower

Celery

Chard

Collard greens

Dandelion greens

Fennel root

Kale

Leeks

Lettuces

Mesclun greens

Mizuna greens

Mustard greens

Onions

Peas (fresh)

Peppers (red, yellow, orange, green)

Radishes (red, black, daikon)

Scallions

Shiitake mushrooms

Sorrel

Spinach

Sprouts (alfalfa, sunflower, clover, radish)

String beans

Summer squashes

Tomatoes

Watercress

White turnips

STARCHY VEGETABLES

Beets

Burdock

Carrots

Celeriac (celery root)

Corn (fresh)

Edamame (fresh soybeans)

Globe artichokes

Jerusalem artichokes

Parsnips

Potatoes

Rutabagas (yellow turnips)

Sweet Potatoes

Winter squashes

Yams

SEA VEGETABLES

Arame

Dulse

Hiziki

Kelp

Nori

Wakame

FRUIT
FRESH

Apples
Apricots
Bananas
Blackberries
Blueberries
Cherries
Clementines
Cranberries
Grapefruits (fresh)
Grapes
Kiwis

Mangoes
Melons
Nectarines
Papayas
Peaches
Pears
Plums
Raspberries
Strawberries
Tangerines

DRIED

Apples
Apricots
Black mission figs
Currants

Dates
Nectarines
Papayas
Prunes

GRAINS, SEEDS, NUTS
GRAINS

Basmati rice
Brown rice
Buckwheat
Jasmine rice
Millet

Quinoa
Sushi rice
Optional: rice cakes

SEEDS—*raw or dry roasted*

Pumpkin
Sesame

Sunflower

NUTS—*raw or dry roasted*

Almonds	Walnuts

PROTEINS AND FATS
PROTEINS

Avocado

Beans—such as adzuki,
  black beans, black-eyed peas,
  cannelini, chick-peas, lima, pinto

Edamame (fresh soybeans)

Fish—such as arctic char, cod,
  haddock, salmon, sardines,
  scrod, tilapia, trout, tuna

Tofu—any consistency

Optional: eggs, miso

FATS

Avocado

Cold-pressed extra-virgin
  olive oil

Flax oil

Optional: unrefined toasted
  sesame oil

CONDIMENTS AND BEVERAGES
CONDIMENTS

Black pepper

Garlic

Ginger

Herbs—fresh or dried,
  such as basil, sage, rosemary, thyme, cilantro,
  parsley, dill

Lemon

Lime

Spices—such as anise,
  cardamom, cayenne,
  cinnamon, cumin

Optional: sea salt, Bragg
  Liquid Aminos

BEVERAGES—*no cold liquids*

Green tea

Herbal tea—such as ginger,
  licorice, and peppermint

Purified water—room
  temperature or warm,
  with lemon optional

SUPPLEMENTS THAT HELP YOUR BODY
CLEANSE

There are many products on the market today to accelerate the cleansing process. While supplements can be beneficial, I don't recommend that people solely rely on them. Along with gently aiding your body's natural healing abilities through disciplined food choices, the purpose of the cleanse is to give you the experience of feeding yourself in a new way. If you're only taking pills or mixing powder drinks, you won't learn much about working with food to keep your body balanced all year long.

In addition to using food to help the body detoxify and cleanse, I do recommend a limited number of optional supplements to facilitate the removal of toxins and the rebuilding of healthy cells. The three optional supplements you may choose to incorporate into your cleanse regimen are a dandelion root tincture, colon cleanser, and a probiotic.

Dandelion root tincture. One of the chief roles of the liver is to filter the blood. For this reason, it's especially important to give the liver an opportunity to release any toxins it has been storing. The bitter green vegetables that grow in early spring—dandelion, arugula, kale, and scallions—stimulate the liver to cleanse. In addition to eating those greens, you can further cleanse the liver by using a dandelion root tincture, which is simply a more potent form of these cleansing bitter greens. A tincture is a concentrated liquid plant extract, which you can dilute in tea or water. You may use a dandelion root tincture, or a tincture that contains dandelion root, burdock, and/or nettles, which you can readily purchase at most natural food stores.

Colon Cleanser. During the cleanse you may also use a fiber or bulking agent to facilitate the elimination of toxins in the colon. I recommend products that include at least some of the following ingredients: psyllium husks or flax seeds, triphila, yellow citrus peel, ginger root, fennel seed, slippery elm bark, bardock root, and chlorophyll.

Probiotic. Finally, I also recommend using a probiotic, which is an active culture that increases the production of healthy bacteria in the gastrointestinal tract. You may purchase either an acidophilus or primadophilus product. Just be sure to use enteric-coated capsules, which can survive the stomach acids and go directly to the intestines.

KEEPING THE DIGESTIVE FIRES BURNING

Cleansing tends to have a cooling effect on the body. With the increase in vegetables and the significant decrease or elimination of animal protein, fats, and complex carbohydrates, your body will be cooler than usual. What this means is that you may become prone to feeling chilled. Feeling cold is one indicator that you need to be extra vigilant about maintaining internal heat. Warmth aids digestion, while cold hinders it. The more you can retain internal heat, the better your digestion will be, and the greater the benefits you will reap from the cleanse. Below are a few simple things you can do to keep the digestive fires burning strong.

Oil. Fat has gotten a very bad reputation in recent years. People today are downright terrified of fat, in just about all of its forms. Of course, the truth is our bodies need fatty acids to work properly, the right kind, that is. When I first work with people, they're shocked by how much olive oil or flax oil I tell them to use; even avocados sound like a decadent treat. At the same time, I help people significantly decrease or eliminate fried foods and refined wheat products. If we have the appropriate kinds and amounts of fat from high-quality oils and vegetable sources such as olive oil, flax oil, canola oil, sesame oil, avocados, almonds, walnuts, and sesame seeds, then our desire for excess amounts of carbohydrates decreases greatly.

Oil helps maintain heat in the system, and is a natural insulator, engendering feelings of warmth and protection. During the cleanse you may use small amounts of flax oil and extra-virgin olive oil (be sure to select cold-pressed olive oil). The amount of oil you use depends on the weather and your personal circumstances. The cooler the weather, the greater your need for oil. Likewise, if you find yourself feeling a bit vulnerable and emotionally raw, then increase the amount of oil you use when roasting vegetables or cooking fish or tofu. If you're cleansing when the weather is warm, use oil more sparingly.

Keep your insides warm with tea. While cleansing, you should drink at least eight to ten cups of liquid a day. Drink hot, warm, or room temperature liquids only: herbal tea, green tea, and spring water. Hot and warm liquids are essential to cleansing, even during the summer months. Remember, during the cleanse we are working toward maximum digestion, absorption, and assimilation, which occurs most optimally when the digestive tract is warm. When you have a stomachache, which makes you feel better: a glass of ice water or a warm cup of tea? Not only is it soothing to hold a warm cup of tea in your hands, but the warm liquid also is more gentle for your body. Cold shocks the stomach and suspends digestive juices, slowing down digestion. Again, because cleansing cools the body, we want to keep the digestive tract warm by consuming room temperature, warm, and hot liquids only.

In my home, I keep a kettle of hot water simmering on the stove all day long. The first thing I do in the morning is put on the kettle, and the last thing I do before going to bed is turn it off. Everyone who comes into my home is offered a cup of tea, and I drink it throughout the day as well. There's nothing that gives you a deeper and more immediate sense of nourishment than holding a warm cup of tea, the steam gently licking your face. Yet people perpetually consume cold beverages. Even in the frigid chill of winter, people start their day with a twenty-four-ounce cup of iced coffee, followed by cans of ice-cold Diet Coke.

I can't stress enough the importance of maintaining warmth in the body throughout the cleanse, as well as during cool or cold times of the year. Travel in the car with hot tea, keep a beautiful clay mug on your desk at work, relax at night with a good book and cup of peppermint tea. Make drinking hot liquids a regular part of your day.

MAKING THE DECISION TO CLEANSE

I use the cleanse as a time to check in with myself. How often do we give something up for fourteen or twenty-one days a year? We give nothing up. This is what's important. You make a commitment to cleanse yourself of all impurities and as a result of that other possibilities emerge. I have awakened something within me that has much more energy than I've ever felt before.

—DREW

SETTING YOUR INTENTION

We can be very disciplined in many areas of our lives. Yet when it comes to food, even the most prudent and responsible people seem to have difficulty limiting what goes into the mouth. Food is our Achilles' heel. While a dictionary informs us that food is nourishment eaten to sustain life, we all know that food has social and personal meanings far more vast than what's needed purely for physical sustenance. Our very childhood, family dynamics, relationships, self-esteem, self-identity, emotions, and health are intricately bound to this mystery called food. I don't know of any other substance so fraught with meaning. It's no wonder then that setting limits on what one eats, even for a short period of time, poses a real challenge to so many people.

The cleanse requires discipline, and the only way for discipline to succeed is if it's accompanied by commitment. When people are clear about their motivation for cleansing, they tend to be more committed to the process and better able to persevere with the discipline. Of course, even a strongly motivated person can still feel very apprehensive about giving up coffee for a few weeks. "How will I possibly function?" we ask ourselves. "Who will I be without coffee?" Fear is a normal part of any journey, particularly one that involves exploring unfamiliar landscapes within oneself. But don't let fear stop you. Feed your intention for change and trust that you will be fully nourished during the cleanse.

As Drew says, the cleanse does ask us to give something up. At first it may feel like you're giving up familiarity, convenience, or comfort. Eventually, everyone who cleanses comes to realize that limiting food choices is just the first step of the process. Ultimately, the cleanse is an opportunity to shed old self-concepts, behaviors, and patterns, and become more who you really are.

Because the cleanse is a rigorous discipline, it's important to be honest about your reasons for wanting to cleanse. Why cleanse? Why now? Perhaps your body has been sending the physical signals that it's time to make significant changes—such as weight gain, insomnia, gastrointestinal disturbances, anxiety—and you're now ready to answer the wake-up call. Maybe you feel that you've gotten far away from your true self and you want to start living in a way that honors your spirit. Possibly discipline is a consistent challenge for you in all areas of your life and you wish to live more responsibly to yourself. This could be a time of transition in your life—changing careers, returning to school, entering a new relationship—and the cleanse is a powerful tool to help you remain steady and strong through your transformation. Take the time to reflect on your own reasons for cleansing. What do you wish to release? Which parts of yourself do you want to strengthen? What aspects of your life need healing at this time?

WHEN IS THE BEST TIME OF YEAR TO CLEANSE?

The best time to start a cleanse is during the transition from one season to the next. Spring and fall are ideal transition times. Because of the transformational qualities of spring and fall, they are optimal times for renewal. I personally cleanse during the summer, when my work schedule is less demanding and the weather is consistently warm. Whether you cleanse during warm or cool weather depends on the season that most invigorates you. Although some people feel the most animated during the bitterest chill of winter, I do not recommend you undertake this cleanse during the cold months of the year. Cold temperatures are simply too extreme for this type of cleanse, and will only result in throwing your body off balance.

Spring: Emerging from the darkness into the light. After many months of darkness and barren gray terrain, I'm always grateful for the crocuses and daffodils, for all the first signs of spring. Life seems to magically reappear after its long winter sleep. Spring is a natural time to cleanse because of the sense of emerging from the darkness, wanting to shed extra layers accumulated during the winter, and activating your body. The young spring shoots make us hopeful for that same renewal within ourselves.

According to Chinese medicine, this also is the time with the greatest liver activity. Detoxifying and cleansing the liver during the spring season supports the gastrointestinal tract and the elimination process, thereby helping you to uncover your fresh new body. Accordingly, many of the vegetables that are available in spring are leafy bitter greens, which also help to flush out your digestive tract, furthering the overall sense of spring renewal. If you live in a cool climate and your body tends to get cold easily, then I caution you against cleansing in the spring.

Summer: Long days of sunshine. During the summer we naturally feel a desire to feed ourselves fresh and light foods. More local produce is available in the markets. The warm weather and long days make it very easy to cleanse during this season. People can be outdoors and active, take vacation time from work. This is personally my favorite time of year to cleanse. If you're like me and depend on sunshine for warmth and relaxation, then the summer may be your ideal cleanse season.

Fall: Harvesting the bounty. The harvest season is also an excellent season to cleanse, when the fruits of the earth are abundant. Even in urban centers, fresh fruits and locally grown vegetables are readily accessible, and we are easily satisfied with the variety of fruits and vegetables that are available. For most of us who've spent a decent portion of our lives attuned to the school calendar, the fall may still represent a time for beginnings or new endeavors. If this is true for you, then harness the energy of new possibilities and cleanse in the fall. If you do choose a fall cleanse, be sure to complete it no later than mid- or late October before the weather becomes too cool.

GEARING UP FOR THE CLEANSE
BEFORE YOU BEGIN A CLEANSE

- Consider cleansing with someone else—a friend, partner or spouse, relative, colleague. It's easier to take on a discipline when you have moral and practical support. Have a regular check-in with your cleanse partner and share meals together.

- Plan to cleanse at a time in your life when your schedule allows you to slow down and fully commit to caring for yourself.

- Create a retreat-like environment for yourself. Establish a framework that allows you the time and physical space to prepare, organize, feed, and pay attention to yourself with more awareness.

- Try a short cleanse at first. If this is your first time cleansing, start with a shorter cleanse to get an idea of how you respond to this discipline physically, emotionally, and spiritually. For example, you can do a three-day cleanse. If you feel great after the three-day cleanse, then continue the last phase for four more days, for a total of seven days. Allow how you feel on the inside to determine the external discipline.

GET RID OF CLUTTER

As you prepare to cleanse, consider using this time to clean your actual house or apartment. Ever notice how good it feels to do a thorough spring-cleaning, purging your closets of unnecessary items, discarding piles of papers, doing a deep cleaning of all those hard to reach places? That's because our external environment has a powerful influence on our internal well-being. I'm always amazed by the number of bags and boxes that come out of my house each year. (And my question is: Where did all of this stuff come from in the first place?) All of this excess in our homes takes up an enormous amount of physical, psychic, and emotional space.

The cleanse process is one of elimination—on all levels. You can harness this energy of rejuvenation and deepen your cleanse experience by literally cleaning out the items in your home you no longer need. In this way, clearing your physical environment reflects your inner work of lightening up and releasing.

Before you begin the cleanse, take time to get rid of the clutter in your home and work environments. Gather up old clothes, toys, books, and household items to donate to a local charity or shelter. Cleaning your home is a wonderful way to prepare for the cleanse. It's a statement of commitment to yourself that the cleanse is important to you and that you are willing to make space in your life for the renewal that is approaching.

CREATE A RETREAT-LIKE ENVIRONMENT FOR YOURSELF

Similar to a meditation retreat, the cleanse is a time to simplify your life, remove yourself from unnecessary distractions, and pay attention to who you really are. As you prepare to cleanse, be aware of the amount of external stimulation in your life. Notice how much time you spend each day watching TV, listening to music, talking on the phone, using a computer, reading the newspaper. Gradually reduce the amount of external stimulation you take in to allow more time to quietly be with yourself.

If you approach the cleanse as an awareness practice, then you will find yourself slowing down and becoming more sensitive as your focus turns inward. Support this valuable gift to yourself by establishing a sacred space in your home and the time to be still. Because you will feel more open, sensitive, and emotionally vulnerable, I caution you to be very deliberate about the forms of media and entertainment you choose to consume during the cleanse. Don't expose yourself to images of violence or overly stimulating movies, TV shows, and books that could trigger intense emotional feelings. Instead, use your free time for creative projects, contemplation, writing in a journal, spending time in nature, reading inspirational texts, or simply resting.

FEED YOURSELF WITH A CALM MIND AND A GRATEFUL HEART

Creating ritual at a meal deeply enhances the nourishment that you receive from your food. Any practice that brings your awareness and gratitude to a meal transforms the experience of eating into the experience of being fed.

Try some of the following practices:

- When you feed yourself, make eating your only activity—avoid eating at your desk, in the car, or on the sofa in front of the TV.
- Set the table with a nice cloth, napkins, a fresh flower, candles.
- Select, write, or improvise a blessing to say before each meal.

- Sit silently for a moment before you begin feeding yourself, calming your mind and opening your body and heart to fully receive the food's nourishment.

- Feed yourself slowly, chewing well, taking the time to really experience the aroma, tastes, and textures of your food.

- Stop eating when you notice that you feel full, yet still have some space in your belly.

PHYSICAL EXERCISE AND BODY BRUSHING

The skin is the largest organ of the body for elimination, and sweating is one way our body naturally releases toxins. Before starting the cleanse, establish a regular exercise routine like walking, jogging, swimming, yoga, bike riding, or working out in the gym, to give your body as many opportunities for cleansing as possible.

Body brushing is another effective and easy way to further eliminate toxins. A daily practice of body brushing stimulates the lymphatic system and encourages the release of toxins through the skin's pores. Take five minutes a day to make this invigorating practice part of your daily routine. You may choose to body brush before or during bathing, in a steam bath, or in a sauna. To body brush, you'll need a loofah sponge, a long-handled natural bristle brush, or a washcloth. If you don't have any of these bath accoutrements, your hands will work just as well.

Begin by brushing the feet and ankles. In long, brisk, sweeping strokes, continue brushing up the entire leg to the abdomen, paying extra attention to stimulating the lymphatic area in the groin region. Then brush from the hands and wrists up the arms and down the chest toward the abdomen, taking the time to thoroughly brush the lymphatic area around the neck, ears, and underarms. Brushing from the extremities toward the center of the body facilitates the removal of toxins from the lymph system through the urine and stools.

FOOD SHOPPING

Because most of the food you will consume is perishable, it's best to buy small quantities of fresh produce every three to four days. When my clients commit to starting a cleanse, they rush out to the natural foods supermarket and purchase almost all of the vegetables and fruits on the cleanse foods list, come home with bulging bags of produce, and stuff them all into the refrigerator. When about half of their beautiful produce spoils before they can eat it, they quickly learn there's no need to hoard all of this food. My clients fear that there won't be enough to eat, or that they won't survive on just vegetables and fruit. Over-shopping is just a natural response to these fears. Until you're familiar with the amounts and kinds of foods you need, it's better to buy too much than to not have enough.

When purchasing produce, try to buy organic when possible. You should also select the produce that has the most vitality. In general, the smaller fruits and vegetables are the most potent. Because their juices are more concentrated than their larger counterparts, this also means the smaller fruits and vegetables are more flavorful. I know this advice runs counter to our cultural conditioning; we've been trained to believe that the bigger item is the better one. But don't let your eyes deceive you. Experiment with different sizes of produce and see for yourself.

PREPARING TO CLEANSE

Breakfast. Start your day with a glass of fresh vegetable juice or fresh-squeezed grapefruit juice. Wait twenty minutes and then have a bowl of fresh seasonal fruit, or plain or vanilla yogurt, hot cereal, or eggs, depending on what fuels you best.

Lunch. Lunch can consist of a fresh salad, soup, steamed or baked vegetables with either a protein (tofu, fish, turkey, chicken, beans) or a grain dish (rice, quinoa, millet, kasha).

Dinner. Similar to lunch, dinner can include a fresh salad, hearty soup, and an abundance of cooked vegetables with either a protein (tofu, fish, turkey, chicken, beans) or a grain dish (rice, quinoa, millet, kasha).

Snacks. Cooked or raw vegetables (red bell pepper, baked sweet potato), almonds, hazelnuts, walnuts, rice cakes with almond butter, yogurt, fresh or dried fruit.

Liquids. Drink eight to ten cups of hot, warm, or room temperature liquid throughout the day, such as herbal tea and spring water.

Paying attention. Take stock of the food and beverages you consume. Be aware of when you feed yourself, why, what you eat, and how much. If it's helpful, write your observations and reflections in a daily journal for the duration of the cleanse.

Ease into the cleanse by making gradual food changes a few weeks *before* your start date. At least one or two weeks before cleansing, eliminate or reduce your consumption of processed foods, soft drinks, refined flour products, dairy, meat, white sugar, alcohol, and caffeine. An immediate change to the cleanse is too much of a shock for your body, and will most likely intensify any cleanse responses you may experience as your body releases toxins. Also begin to gently ease your digestion through food combining practices (see page 90) if you aren't already following these guidelines.

When you replace toxin-forming foods with simpler and purer ones, at first toxins circulate more freely through the bloodstream before being eliminated through the intestines. People generally feel the most intense physical and emotional reactions to the sudden release of toxins during the first phase of the cleanse. This is why a preparation period is so crucial. The only way to lessen the intensity of these normal yet challenging responses is by gradually preparing your body in the weeks leading up to your cleanse.

Use this preparation time to clean and organize your kitchen, refrigerator, cabinets, and pantry. I know, sometimes the back of the refrigerator looks as though it's a storage unit for your children's science projects. But take heart and throw away last Thanksgiving's moldy jar of cranberry sauce and other containers of spoiled food that have been hibernating in the back of your shelves. Toss out half-eaten containers of ice cream and give away or dispose of foods that may tempt you during the cleanse, like frozen bagels, macaroni and cheese, crackers, cookies, corn chips. If you live with other people, consider designating a cabinet, shelf, or area of the refrigerator for your cleanse foods.

Also try to organize your family and work schedules so that you have more time to shop, prepare food, and focus on yourself.

Let your family know what you're planning to do, and solicit the appropriate support from them. That's not to say that you won't get questions and raised eyebrows when you tell them your plans. Just take a deep breath and explain your intentions. If possible, also try to keep social engagements to a minimum, particularly those that center around eating. Regardless of the length of time you have chosen to cleanse, you will need this extra support from the very beginning.

PHASE ONE: VEGETABLES AND FRUIT

- Any combination of vegetables (including avocado)
- Fruit eaten alone

Upon rising. Probiotic and colon cleanser (see page 123), glass of water or fresh vegetable juice.

Breakfast. Lightly cooked vegetables *or* a bowl of fruit. Cup of tea with dandelion root tincture (see page 122). **Suggestion:** Try a beautiful bowl of pear, apple, and banana slices with a sprinkling of currants. Or have stewed apples with cinnamon. If you feel unfocused and foggy or experience an immediate drop of energy after eating fruit, you would be better served by eating vegetables for breakfast, such as hash browns (see recipe page 279) with avocado slices.

Lunch and dinner. Vegetable soup, fresh salad, and a variety of vegetable dishes, which can be raw, steamed, sautéed, baked, roasted, or broiled. Cup of tea with dandelion root tincture.

Snacks. Cooked or raw vegetables, sea vegetables, fresh or dried fruit, rice cakes if needed.

Liquids. Drink eight to ten cups of hot, warm, or room temperature liquids throughout the day, such as herbal tea and spring water. Three of those cups should include dandelion root tincture (see page 122).

Paying attention. Try preparing a meal with acute awareness of all your senses. Wash, chop, and stir paying attention to the smells, colors, textures, and shapes of your food. Notice how smells expand and color and texture change as you heat, steam, boil, or bake your food. Finally, when it's time to eat, allow the food to nourish you through all of your senses.

See page 118 for a list of cleanse foods and page 187 for cleanse recipes.

During the cleanse, you will feed yourself highly nutritious foods that are easy to digest and help you eliminate the excess from your body. In addition, you will consume foods that give you the most energy and have the least toxic effect on your body. The foods that give us the most energy while creating balance in the body are the green, chlorophyll-rich vegetables, hearty root vegetables, and sea vegetables. These are your primary food sources during the cleanse. Don't worry, this doesn't mean that you only eat salads day in and day out. While cleansing, you're free to have an unlimited amount of vegetables. Just make sure you have a balance of starchy root vegetables and leafy green vegetables.

The highest concentration of chlorophyll is found in green,

leafy vegetables such as kale, watercress, chard, collard greens, and mesclun greens. The deeper the green, the better. Not only do these greens provide roughage to help the body gently eliminate excess matter, but the chlorophyll also detoxifies the body's organs and cleanses the blood. In addition to leafy green vegetables, the other important foods for cleansing are the mineral-rich root and sea vegetables. Minerals—such as calcium, sodium, magnesium, and iron—are essential to the optimal functioning of our bodies. Because the daily American diet contains so few minerals, most people today rely on taking vitamins as their only source of these vital nutrients. During the cleanse, you will explore mineral-rich food sources such as root vegetables that absorb minerals through the soil and sea vegetables that are power-packed with minerals from the ocean (see page 97). I encourage you to explore the world of these delicious and healthful vegetables, particularly if they are new to you.

While you may consume an unlimited quantity of vegetables, you do need to exercise caution when it comes to fruit. Sweet, juicy, and succulent, fruit truly is the gift of the gods. Limiting your fruit consumption isn't meant to deny you this sweet pleasure, but to protect you from cleansing too rapidly. Because fruit is digested so quickly (approximately twenty to thirty minutes), it tends to accelerate the cleansing process. This may seem like a benefit, but you should be cautious about how quickly you engage in any cleanse.

Detoxifying too quickly can be overwhelming as well as discouraging. When toxins enter the bloodstream so quickly, reactions sometimes occur, such as headaches, nausea, joint and muscle pains, and emotional irritability. These reactions are bound to happen in the cleansing process, but it's better to control their intensity during the early stages of the cleanse when your body is adjusting to major digestive changes. In general, limit your fruit intake to about twenty percent of the bulk of food you consume in a day. If you're uncertain about the appropriate quantity of fruit, just remember that less is better.

PHASE TWO:
GRAINS, SEEDS, AND NUTS

- Grains combined with any vegetables (except avocado)
- Seeds or nuts combined with any vegetables (except avocado)
- Grains, seeds, and nuts should be eaten separately

Upon rising. Probiotic and colon cleanser (see page 123), glass of water or fresh vegetable juice.

Breakfast. Lightly cooked vegetables *or* cooked grains *or* a bowl of fruit. Cup of tea with dandelion root tincture (see page 122). **Suggestion:** Many people enjoy the same breakfast meal every day while cleansing. If you find a meal that fuels you well and doesn't bore you, continue to eat it for the duration of the cleanse. Otherwise, experiment with different combinations of vegetables and/or grain dishes. For instance, consider starting your day with a bowl of hearty vegetable soup and a bowl of quinoa.

Lunch and dinner. Grain *or* baked vegetables, steamed vegetables, vegetable soup, fresh salad. Cup of tea with dandelion root tincture. **Suggestion:** Separate the starchy vegetables from your grain meal so that you don't have baked squash and rice at the same time, for example. If you feed yourself grains for lunch, have a small bowl of rice, salad, and a stir-fry medley of broccoli, kale, shiitake mushrooms, and onions. For dinner that night have a salad, vegetable soup, and roasted beets and yellow turnips.

Bedtime (optional). Probiotic and colon cleanser (see page 123).

Snacks. Cooked or raw vegetables, sea vegetables, rice cakes, seeds or nuts, fresh or dried fruit.

Liquids. Drink eight to ten cups of hot, warm, or room temperature liquids throughout the day, such as herbal tea and spring water. Three of those cups should include dandelion root tincture (see page 122).

Paying attention. Have a "no media meal." Feed yourself a meal without the distractions of the TV, a newspaper, your computer, a book. Give yourself plenty of time to enjoy your food. After the meal, sit quietly for a few moments before you get up from the table. Feel the deep satisfaction from the nourishment that's just entered your body.

See page 118 for a list of cleanse foods and page 187 for cleanse recipes.

In the second phase of the cleanse, you can have one to two grain meals per day, depending on your individual needs. The grains phase of the cleanse tends to be highly individual, varying from person to person. For some people, grains are a wonderful source of fuel; for others, even whole grains can keep them stuck in their carbohydrate addiction. How do you know where you belong on this spectrum? I recommend that you experiment with grains during your cleanse preparation time. Prepare a grain and vegetable meal—such as rice and sautéed vegetables—and then pay careful attention to how you feel one, two, and three hours later. Do you crave more carbohydrates or sugar? Do you feel a little drop in energy, or is the grain a strong fuel that keeps you going for a few hours? If you find that it does fuel you, then you will have no problem with grains during the cleanse.

On the other hand, if grains cause you to have low energy or you have the instant craving to consume more carbohydrates, then I would recommend you modify your grain consumption on the cleanse. Here are a few options for people with grain sensitivities: Eat only a small portion of grain each day; eat grain every other day; or bypass the grains phase altogether and divide your cleanse into a vegetables/fruit phase and a protein phase. The season in which you're cleansing is another factor to consider. In general, when the weather is cool, grain will help you retain body heat and keep you feeling grounded. In warm or hot weather, you won't necessarily need a lot of grain.

During this phase we also introduce seeds and nuts. The seeds and nuts I recommend are sunflower seeds, pumpkin seeds, sesame seeds, almonds, and walnuts. During this second phase of the cleanse, we are still trying to support simple digestion. For this reason, seeds and nuts should not be eaten in the same meal with grains, because the protein and carbohydrate combination complicates digestion. If you feed yourself almonds or pumpkin seeds, have them as far apart from your grain meal as possible. Eat them as a snack or part of your vegetable meal.

When purchasing seeds and nuts, it's best to buy them raw and organic, if possible. Just a word of caution about buying roasted seeds and nuts. While they may be tasty, these seeds and nuts usually contain high quantities of added salt and tend to be roasted in poor quality oils. If you like roasted seeds and nuts, you can easily roast them yourself. Dry roasting seeds and nuts enhances their flavor, adds crunch, and makes them easier to digest. To oven roast, preheat the oven to 350°. Place the seeds or nuts on an ungreased baking sheet, lower the heat to 300°, and bake for 8–12 minutes. You may also pan roast seeds and nuts on the stovetop. Cast iron skillets work best. Place the seeds or nuts in the pan over medium-high heat, stirring regularly with a wooden spoon until they are lightly toasted and fragrant. Be careful, the pumpkin seeds will pop! For a little variety, you may add sea salt, Bragg Liquid Aminos, dulse granules, or crumbled wakame.

Additionally, almonds are excellent when soaked. Soaking almonds increases their digestibility and brings out their sweet flavor. To soak almonds, place a small amount in a bowl and cover with water. Let the almonds soak overnight. Change the water in the morning and refrigerate. To avoid fermenting, it's best to soak almonds in small quantities—as many as you plan to consume in one or two days.

I frequently hear from people that the crunchiness of seeds and nuts often sparks the addictive pattern of wanting more. They are small and easy to grab, so you need to be cautious about how you use them. If you find yourself frequently snacking on seeds and nuts, then remove the seeds and nuts or be very disciplined about how much you consume. Because they will cause some congestion within the digestive tract, at most have only two to three tablespoons of seeds, or approximately fifteen to twenty almonds per day.

PHASE THREE: PROTEIN

- Protein combined with any vegetables
- Protein should be eaten separately from grains, seeds, and nuts

Upon rising. Probiotic and colon cleanser (see page 123), glass of water or fresh vegetable juice.

Breakfast. Lightly cooked vegetables *or* cooked grains *or* a protein dish *or* a bowl of fruit. Cup of tea with dandelion root tincture (see page 122).

Lunch and dinner. Grain *or* tofu *or* fish *or* beans, steamed and/or baked vegetables, vegetable soup, fresh salad. Cup of tea with dandelion root tincture. **Suggestion:** The protein meal should not include grain, but a starchy vegetable can be very satisfying. Try having broiled or poached fresh fish with baked squash drizzled with olive oil and garlic, accompanied by a salad with a variety of vegetables.

Bedtime (optional). Probiotic and colon cleanser (see page 123).

Snacks. Cooked or raw vegetables, sea vegetables, rice cakes, seeds or nuts, fresh or dried fruit.

Liquids. Drink eight to ten cups of hot, warm, or room temperature liquids throughout the day, such as herbal tea and spring water. Three of those cups should include dandelion root tincture (see page 122).

Paying attention. Alone, or in the company of others who would like to try this experience with you, create an entire meal as an awareness practice. As you feed yourself, be aware of all the movements you make in the process of eating, from lifting your fork to chewing and swallowing. Notice the aroma, flavors, textures, and consistency of your food. Fully experience each mouthful. Notice the difference in sensation when you have soup or drink something compared to eating solid foods. Make your awareness so subtle that you can actually feel your food travel down into your stomach. At what point do you cease to experience your food? At what point does your food become you?

See page 118 for a list of cleanse foods and page 187 for cleanse recipes.

Aside from fats, proteins are one of the most complex matters for our bodies to digest. Following the guidelines of food combining and to support easy digestion, proteins can be consumed with vegetables, but not with grains. Your protein meal will consist of a portion of tofu, fish, or beans, accompanied by an array of vegetables. Although they also are complex carbohydrates, for the purposes of the cleanse, beans are included with proteins because they are more difficult to digest than grains.

In general, six to eight ounces of protein a day is sufficient for most people during the cleanse (the equivalent of a small piece of salmon). Like the grains phase, this phase also varies for people. Some people require more protein, particularly if they are very physically active, have a demanding schedule, or are experiencing a lot of stress in their life. Others may choose to have less protein or to feed themselves protein every other day. Rely on your own energy levels as a guideline for how much grain or protein you need.

This phase of the cleanse is when we transition to a more inclusive way of feeding ourselves. With the reintroduction of protein, this final stage gently brings your body out of the cleansing modality without the risk of shocking your system. The third phase of the cleanse is the most similar to our normal way of feeding ourselves. For this reason, it's an excellent opportunity to see how you can feed yourself plenty of nourishment—from proteins and grains to vegetables and fruits—but in a cleaner way that keeps your energy strong and balanced. If you feel good feeding yourself this way, then continue this phase for as long as you wish.

COMMON CLEANSE EXPERIENCES

The cleanse is empowering. I realized I could do a twenty-one-day cleanse and come out the other end. People told me I glowed, and I did. I still have that glow, especially when I'm adhering to eating cleanly. Sure, I can put bad stuff into my body, but I won't feel good. And I can quickly say to myself, "Okay, this isn't working. I have to go back and do what I was doing." That's a tool I can rely on for the rest of my life. It's like creating solid building blocks for your house. If you take care of your house, it will stand you in good stead. It may grow old, but it can grow old to the best of its abilities.

—EMILY

People often cleanse because they want to improve their health, feel mentally clear, and have more energy. These are wonderful aspirations, but to arrive at this balanced and energized state, sometimes we have to go through challenging physical and emotional experiences first. That's why this is called a *cleanse*. But people usually forget this when they're dealing with headaches, skin rashes, or exhaustion. We have a vision of how we want to feel at the end of the cleanse, but there's no other way to get there than to go through it.

By cleansing, you consciously give your body permission to eliminate toxins and old matter that already exist within the system. Cleanse responses, both physical and emotional, are a normal part of the process, and you should be prepared to experience them to a certain degree. Essentially, a cleanse response is just an intensification of a preexisting emotional or physical condition. Responses can take the form of rashes, scaly skin, headaches, constipation, diarrhea, fatigue, itchiness, an unsettled stomach, anger, melancholy, or changes in the menstrual cycle, as well as other responses. If people experience difficult cleanse responses, I always recommend they eat more vegetables, because vegetables ease the reaction. As long as you get enough exercise, rest, and eat plenty of vegetables, then letting the body eliminate toxins is an essential part of the cleansing process.

The first phase of the cleanse is the period where digestion is the easiest and the body has more energy for elimination. The greatest amount of toxins will be deposited into the bloodstream during this phase. If you are going to experience a cleanse response, it usually will occur during this first phase, particularly if you normally consume a lot of caffeine, wheat, or sugar. Although symptoms like headaches, dizziness, lack of focus, and lethargy may not feel very pleasant, they are very good. These symptoms indicate that your body is doing exactly what you've asked it to do and is releasing what's excess and unnecessary.

If you experience a cleanse response, it's important to respond to it with a gentle attitude of nonattachment. Don't resist the response. Pay attention to it but also know that in time it will change. Nourish yourself extra well by getting plenty of rest, taking hot baths, exercising gently, spending time with loved ones, and insulating yourself from unnecessary stimulation. Eliminating toxins is an essential and natural part of the cleanse. It's also an opportunity to learn how to communicate with your body. In time, you will notice the kinds and amounts of food that trigger physical and emotional responses for you. As you learn to trust your body's wisdom, its process, and its sense of timing, you will open to greater opportunities for transformation and healing.

While cleansing you can expect considerable changes in how your body eliminates. When digestion is easier and the body can readily absorb nutrients through the intestinal walls, stools are eliminated more frequently, easily, and completely. For many people, this comes as a great relief. On the cleanse, you can expect to eliminate a meal anytime from eight to twelve hours after it has been consumed. By contrast, a person with blocked intestines—who regularly eats processed foods, refined wheat products, meat, and dairy and gets little exercise—usually eliminates a meal anytime from twenty-four to seventy-two hours later.

Use the cleanse as an opportunity to observe your eliminations to better understand how your body is digesting particular foods you have eaten. If there is a preexisting condition toward constipation or intermittent diarrhea, you may initially experience an increase in these body responses before they improve. Be patient and trust the process. Even during the relatively short time of the cleanse, the body can respond to changes in one's diet very quickly, which is reflected in better elimination. You will know when digestion is improving. Your body will feel lighter and more balanced.

INTEGRATING THE CLEANSE INTO EVERYDAY LIFE

If you've ever been on a retreat of any kind—meditation, yoga, art, or music—you know that a few days or hours before you leave, it's very common to feel anxious about returning to your normal life. "How can I maintain the peaceful equilibrium I found on retreat," you wonder to yourself. "How can I continue to be as creative as I've been during this past week?" Self-growth and development are relatively easy when you are on a retreat. The hard part is going home. Retreats can be a wonderful time for a jump start or tune-up, but I find that the real work is integrating what you've learned into your daily reality and maintaining a lifestyle that fosters continued growth. As the cleanse draws to a close, you may have the overwhelming sense of *now what?* Without the structure of the cleanse to guide you in your food choices, what will happen?

For most of us, the discipline of the cleanse is too restrictive to maintain all the time. Post-cleanse, some people continue a five-day-a-week discipline, where they more or less follow the principles of the third phase of the cleanse. On the weekends, they are more relaxed with the discipline. Another approach is to do a mini-cleanse one day a week, where you eat mostly vegetables and some fruit. Monday is a great day for this "green day" because it creates the focus for the rest of the week. You may wish to make an annual cleanse part of your yearly rhythm. Another practical approach to keeping yourself balanced is to make sure you have enough time to prepare and plan ahead. One client told me that she learned from the cleanse to "make food a priority instead of a last-minute scramble." By making food a priority, you are in fact making it a priority to nourish yourself.

The cleanse gives you an opportunity to find out more about your body and how you feel when you feed yourself according to the cleanse principles. What foods worked well for you on the cleanse? Which will you continue to have on a regular basis? Some clients want to continue eating a greater quantity and variety of vegetables, including green salads, seasonal squash, and kale. Others have told me they want to eat in tune with the seasons. Many people make the commitment to continue eating less refined foods, sugar, wheat, and salt. Reflect on what you learned from your own experience and continue to eat the foods that fuel you the best.

In addition to a better understanding of their bodies, the cleanse gives people a taste of a deeper source of energy, vitality, purpose, and the momentum to move in new directions in their lives. When you clear out the excess in your body, you remove the blocks that impede your entire physical, emotional, mental, and spiritual system. With the body lighter and functioning more cleanly, you recognize that you are not merely a body that needs to be maintained: You are a spiritual being with a purpose here on earth. This taste can be life altering because you will want to return to that place within yourself regularly. Once you've touched your essence, you will want to come back.

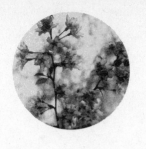

PART THREE

AWAKENING YOUR SPIRIT

7

DISCIPLINE: THE ROOT OF FREEDOM

The spiritual path is made up of disciplined practice, as regular as a heartbeat.

—*Swami Chidvilasananda* (GURUMAYI), The Yoga of Discipline

For as long as I can remember, my daughter has had an affinity for everything Chinese—language, food, stories, movies, people. When she was ten she asked if she could study Chinese language and culture at a nearby school. For some kids it's piano lessons, for others it's karate. For my daughter, it was Chinese school every Saturday morning for seven years. Last spring her class held a graduation celebration, and the students sang, read poems, played music, and gave speeches. When it was Yasemin's turn on stage, I was completely amazed. There was my daughter, reading an essay she had written in what everyone said was perfect Mandarin. I glanced around the auditorium at all of the Chinese faces and quickly realized that I was the only one who couldn't understand a word she said.

As you may realize, Chinese is not an easy language to learn. While my daughter has a natural talent for languages, she couldn't have learned without regular practice. She didn't just study Chinese once a week; she made time for it regularly. What's more, I didn't hound her to study; she did it of her own will. Of course, practice isn't limited to the study of languages. All acquired skills require practice and frequent repetition. That's simply how humans learn. For practice to amount to anything it has to be steady, "as regular as a heartbeat," as the Hindu spiritual teacher Gurumayi puts it. If you take one ballroom dance class, you may learn a few moves to impress your friends the next time you're at a party. But the Fred Astaires of the world train regularly for years. When they sweep across the floor—or dance up the sides of walls—all those years of sore muscles and blistered feet and dedicated practice have turned into precision, grace, and ease.

Even though practice is the principal mode by which we acquire skills, it doesn't mean that it comes easily for us. Practice requires discipline. For a marathon runner, discipline means getting up every morning and running before going to work. It means running through the rain and wind, as well as on the glorious bright blue mornings. And sometimes it means saying no to a night out with friends so you can get out of bed the next day and start all over again. Discipline challenges and tests us every step of the way. With discipline, there's no halfway. You can't have one foot in the door and one foot out and expect to make strides with your chosen discipline.

If it weren't for discipline, doctors wouldn't make it through medical school; musicians couldn't play symphonies; farmers wouldn't rise at the crack of dawn to cultivate the food we need to survive. When it comes to eating, so many of us lose the backbone of discipline that supports us going to school, raising families, contributing to our communities, succeeding professionally, and in so many other areas of our lives. It's an interesting phenomenon. One woman I work with told me that until she began to practice transformational nourishment, dieting and the fat content of food was the only awareness she had of eating. Unfortunately, her story is more the norm than the exception. Today, our principal relationship to food is either one of denial and deprivation or total indulgence.

Clients keep telling me they are tired of stuffing their faces all the time. People are fed up with eating on the go, rushing through their meals, eating in front of the computer and TV, grabbing whatever's available, and eating way past the point of comfort. It would be great if we could hang For Sale signs on our bodies and simply move somewhere else. But of course we can't. This is our one body. This is our life. Instead of moving out, try moving in by providing yourself with a loving discipline. Only you can take care of the single most precious gift you've been given in this lifetime: you.

BECOMING A DISCIPLE
OF YOUR SPIRIT

Deep down, many of us yearn to stop the food roller coaster and regain control over our lives. Dieting simply doesn't do it. When people come to see me, they've usually tried a whole host of diets, which has only left them feeling exasperated, in despair, and alienated from their bodies. Dieting is big business in this country. According to the American Dietetic Association, each year more than half of all Americans try to either lose weight or maintain a recent weight loss. The Atkins diet book has been on *The New York Times* best-seller list for many years. Some people can muster their inner resources, their willpower, to stick to a diet for a period of time. But as the statistics show, the results usually are short-lived.

Why do so many people struggle with diets? As well intentioned and sensible as some food programs are, most of them tend to keep us trapped in the physical realm of existence, ignoring the deeper spiritual hunger that exists within each of us. Our spirit's hunger ultimately propels our growth, creativity, desire to learn, and to be of service in the world. I have come to understand that unless we are motivated to nourish this place within ourselves, regular disciplined food choices will continue to evade us.

Maybe in your heart of hearts you recognize this yearning to feed your spirit. Perhaps you sense that life has a deeper purpose and you want to begin living each day in accordance with that vision. If this rings true for you, then you know how it feels to want to live passionately and in service to your spirit. When we are motivated to live a life of spirit, then feeding ourselves ceases to be such a dramatic struggle. From this motivation, we can harness our inner discipline, the willingness to endure no matter how difficult it may be.

The word *discipline* comes from the Latin for *disciple*. If we think of nourishment as a discipline then we see it's just one way to become a disciple of your own spirit. Other disciplines serve the same purpose—from prayer to meditation, yoga, writing, music, and martial arts. And perhaps one or some of these practices work best for you. The gift of nourishment is that we have to do it every day. We just don't say: "Well, I don't feel like feeding myself today. I think I'll take the day off!" Each time we feed ourselves is an opportunity to practice self-love, compassion, and reverence for our spiritual nature.

The willingness to engage in this discipline doesn't mean that a lifetime's worth of patterns will change overnight. No, I can assure you that the myriad food choices, pressured schedules, and emotional associations will all be there tomorrow. That's okay. Be compassionate with yourself no matter where you are in your relationship to feeding yourself. Even switching from drinking soft drinks to spring or purified water is a powerful change. Water is the essence of life: Our earth is comprised mostly of water; we ourselves are made of 90 percent water. We have to get in the practice of seeking out whole and alive sources for what enters our mouths. As simplistic as this may seem, even water makes a difference. When you pay attention to feeding yourself, the doors of awareness open in all areas of your life. Take a deep breath and remember that like most things really worth having, nourishment isn't a quick fix but a long-term commitment to yourself.

CLEARING THE EXCESS

"Fill your bowl to the brim, and it will spill," says Lao Tzu in the *Tao Te Ching*. When the bowl spills over, that's excess. Now imagine that our bodies are that bowl that's been filled too much, where does the excess spill over? It's easy to think of physical excess only as extra weight, but excess can take many forms: mucus, yeast, cholesterol, plaque, caffeine, sugar, even stress and anxiety. All forms of excess create imbalances in our bodies, which directly affects our emotional and spiritual states of consciousness. We starve our spirits when we live lives of excess—from excess processed foods and overconsumption to the pace at which we live and the stress we endure. It's very difficult to feel focused and motivated when your body is so burdened just by trying to maintain its biological functioning.

Excess usually is an indicator of an addiction to the substance that's creating the excess condition in the first place. If you can't think straight before drinking your morning cup of coffee, then chances are there's an excess of caffeine in your system. We mostly crave foods that are already in excess within our bodies. Wheat and sugar are two ingredients that typically cause trouble for most people. Wheat and sugar are everywhere you turn, and in readily available forms—muffins, bread products, doughnuts, pizza, sandwiches, cake, cookies, candy, frozen dairy treats, soft drinks, even in the now-popular energy bars. On and on. And they taste good to us, so good that they're perpetually calling us to have more.

Many of my clients agonize over the candy bowl at the office. I'm not sure when the phenomenon of the candy bowl started, but it seems to be a common fixture in the workplace today. "I can hear the candy bowl calling my name all day long," Sadie told me. "It's a background noise I can ignore for most of the day, and then it gets really clever and persistent. 'Take a break,' it says, 'you deserve a little reward.'"

When we're at, or past, the point of hunger and haven't prepared food for ourselves in advance, of course it's easy to grab the nearest thing available. Unfortunately, these quick-fix foods tend to be highly refined, made with lots of sugar, oil, salt, or wheat, and don't really satisfy our hunger. They fill us up without fueling us up.

If you eat quick-fix foods on a regular basis, they most likely will lead to physical and emotional addictions, where we physically crave those foods and believe our happiness depends on eating them. On the other hand, vital essence foods don't have that addictive quality; you feed yourself, and then you feel satisfied. Have you ever felt midnight compulsions to raid the refrigerator for leftover kale and salmon? Cookies, cereal and milk, or ice cream are probably more like it. Vital essence foods simply don't call you to overindulge.

When the body can no longer withstand the excesses, it will let you know. A response like a sinus or yeast infection, even arthritis, can be the body's way of saying, "Enough!" Each body is different, but the body's voice generally remains the same throughout your life. Excess conditions have the tendency to affect the weaker part of one's system. For example, if you were prone to stomachaches as a child, as an adult you most likely will have a propensity for gastrointestinal reactions if there's excess in your body.

Excess in the body is just like having a cluttered home. Some people can live quite happily and productively amidst a lot of clutter, but I believe that few of us truly thrive in those conditions. You know how good it feels to clean your closets, recycle stacks of old papers and magazines, and give away clothes you haven't worn for years. Your home feels lighter, clearer; it's a place where you actually want to spend time. Because our external home is such a powerful metaphor for our *internal* home, I always suggest that people do a spring-cleaning before they begin a cleanse. Clearing the excess creates more space, literally and metaphorically, so that we have more room to grow, change, and consider possibilities we may never have allowed ourselves to think about before.

ROAMING FREE IN A SMALL MEADOW

At a New Year's Eve party I attended there was a wonderful dark chocolate cake, freshly baked at a European bakery that morning. It was so delicious, I decided to have a second slice. Just as I was putting the cake on my plate, a friend approached me and said, "You're having a second piece of cake!" Obviously my friend had been watching me and was shocked that I, the nourishment consultant, was taking another helping of sugar, wheat, and butter. "Yes," I said, "I'm having two pieces of chocolate cake. Would you like some?"

I don't have chocolate cake every day because I know my

body does not respond well to those ingredients. But I will have cake once or twice a year, and really relish it when I do. An occasional slice of good-quality cake at a party won't cause any problems, but cake on a regular basis would wreak havoc on my system. I suddenly would start craving more cake, and my thoughts would turn to wanting that cake every day. Also, my digestion and elimination would become irregular, my energy would drop, and I wouldn't have the same attention I need to focus on my work, clients, husband, children, as well as my inner growth and development.

In this country, our desiring nature is very well fed. Whatever you want you can pretty much give yourself at any time. *I feel like a piece of chocolate. I need a cup of coffee. I would love a plate of pasta, a large plate of pasta. It's such a hot day, I need a frozen yogurt.* Day after day. We spend lifetimes feeding this desiring nature. In some spiritual traditions this is called "monkey mind." I think this term is very appropriate. Our wanting is an incessant internal chatter: "I need this. I want that. Let's do this. Let's do that." Indeed, it is as though we are jumping from one tree branch to another. In developing the perseverance to maintain a discipline, someone needs to be in control. But who is in control? Who can say to the monkey: "Stop"?

To feed ourselves in a way that respects our inherent need for balance, we have to set limits for ourselves. Limiting our choices quite naturally helps us tame the monkey and stay more balanced. With millions of food products available to us at all times, how do we begin to make sense out of what to feed ourselves? If you've ever eaten at a restaurant with a particularly large menu, then you know it's much more difficult to decide what to order than if you had only one page of choices. Variety is wonderful, but the volume of food choices that are all around simply overwhelms us. To make matters worse, the quality of these choices often is questionable.

Creating limits doesn't mean that we deny or starve ourselves, though at first it may feel that way. When Caitlin joined one of my cleanse groups she was panicked to learn that she would have to give up her main comfort food for the two weeks of the cleanse. Caitlin loved bread, all kinds of bread. She ate it every day, with each meal and even between meals. She joked that she would have been perfectly content to live in prison on a diet of bread and water. "I never thought I could give up bread," she told our group at the end of the two weeks. "Where would that leave me? Well, where it left me was free from the prison I was inhabiting. What I learned from the cleanse was that I was already in prison, and that I could set myself free."

Instead of living in servitude to our cravings, we can nourish our bodies and spirits by limiting our choices and making purposeful decisions about food. In this way, food can help us find the internal balance and harmony we all strive for. So you see, there's a choice. We can exist in a large field but be tethered all the time, or in a smaller meadow where we are free to roam.

8

LIVING YOUR RHYTHM

If people can be clear and calm, heaven and earth will come to them.

—LAO TZU, Tao Te Ching

How do you feel after a bad night's sleep? How about a few sleepless nights in a row? What happens when you skip a meal? What about when you're late for work and have to spend the rest of the day trying to catch up? Or you get a call at the office that your child is sick and needs to get picked up early from school?

Our lives are made up of finely choreographed rhythms. Rhythms are so crucial to our well-being and sense of feeling secure in our lives and the world that we instantly feel off kilter if only one of our basic rhythms is out of balance. In fact, we don't pay much attention to these rhythms while they're humming along smoothly, maintaining a consistent pattern. If you have any doubts about the significance of rhythm in your life, then ask yourself how you honestly feel when your sleep is disrupted or you are constipated for a few days.

We also notice when natural cycles are out of sync. Living in New England, people get concerned when the winter is unusually mild and there's little snowfall. All you hear is talk about global warming trends. "Something is off," people will say forlornly, putting away their unused cross-country skis for another year.

Rhythms are our lifeline. They keep us connected to our bodies as well as to our families, friends, vocations, culture, spiritual life, and nature. The rhythms of the seasons. The cycle of the earth around the sun. The phases of the moon. Every year a tree acquires a new ring. For women each month represents a cycle of fertility. We learn the rhythms of life and death from the plant world; in the winter trees are bare, in the spring and summer they bud and fruit. Elaborate spiritual and cultural rituals have been created to formalize and revere the sacredness of our most important life rhythms, from birth to coming of age, marriage, old age, and death. Indeed, as it's written in Ecclesiastes, "To everything there is a season, and a time to every purpose under the heaven."

Natural rhythms are supportive and nurturing. They keep us aligned to ourselves and connected to other people, nature, the divine. For millennia, the rhythms of a people emerged to support that population in all cycles of their lives—from the harvest and hunting to significant life passages and spiritual contemplation and rites.

Unfortunately, many of our contemporary rhythms fail to nourish us in these important ways. Our rhythms are in danger of becoming restricted to the very small and isolating pattern of a forty- or fifty-hour workweek with weekends, holidays, and two vacations a year. In our culture, many of our personal, familial, and societal rhythms have been imposed from a market-driven mentality. Our world today is faster than ever before. Fast machines, fast computers, fast modes of transportation have created fast lives, in which we eat fast foods. We eat quickly, too, and on the go or while multitasking at the office. Digestive disturbances are so common today, there's a whole aisle in the drugstore devoted to easing their painful symptoms. While digestive problems point to real physical imbalances, I also see them as an important metaphor. People today simply cannot digest their lives. One of the ironies of our age is that the pace of life has never been quicker, yet we have less time available to us.

When the outer rhythms conflict with one's natural inner rhythms, it creates a stressful environment for all of us—people, animals, and the earth. "It's becoming apparent that some of our major physiological and psychological ills may be a result of being out of synch with environmental time," writes Layne Redmond in her exploration of the history of rhythm from a female perspective, *When the Drummers Were Women*. Redmond goes on to quote anthropologist Edward T. Hall, who suggests that "it is the tension between the internal clocks and the clock on the wall that causes so much of the stress in today's world. . . . We have now constructed an entire complex system of schedules, manners, and expectations to which we are trying to adjust ourselves, when, in reality, it should be the other way around."

Our natural rhythms are much slower than the pace at which we live today. We all complain about not having enough time. We don't have enough time for our children, spouses, friends, hobbies, to exercise, relax, travel. We don't have time for ourselves. When people approach the end of their lives, the most common regret voiced is not having spent enough time with loved ones. In the end, how we use our time is more essential than the money or material objects we leave behind.

Most people I've worked with are convinced that they don't have time to shop or cook. Yet some of these same people quite capably complete cleanses where they prepare all of their meals themselves for three weeks. My clients didn't discover a magical extra hour in the day. Because feeding themselves became a priority, they found ways to shift their external rhythms to accommodate their internal rhythms. Ultimately, this creates the sense of having more time—and freedom and control—in your life because you're living in tune to a rhythm that truly nourishes you.

We can't nourish ourselves if we don't learn how to listen to and honor our own rhythms. This doesn't mean you have to "drop out of society" or build a self-sufficient house "off the grid." Living your rhythm isn't a utopian ideal or a romanticization of a simpler past. Living your rhythm is essential to your health, happiness, and overall well-being.

What is our natural rhythm? All the information we need to learn our natural rhythm is at our fingertips—and in our arms and legs and kidneys and spleen. . . . Even if you have two left feet and consider yourself the most uncoordinated person you've ever met, take heart knowing that your body is a finely tuned rhythmic instrument. Our bodies beat to the regular pulse of our biological functioning. Known as *biorhythms*, these rhythms keep our hearts pumping, oxygen circulating, and nutrients flowing to our cells. The body's regular rhythms also keep us perpetually in the process of renewing ourselves. As Elson M. Haas, M.D., notes in *Staying Healthy with the Seasons*, "New blood cells are made daily and the total blood is replaced every 120 days, cells of the soft tissues are replaced every 12 weeks, and bone cells about every 12 months. The oldest cells in the body are supposedly no more than seven years old."

What's more, the same cellular rhythm that exists in me also exists in you. Each tiny cell maintains a steady rhythm of knowing when to accept nutrients and when to eliminate waste matter, when to divide, and when to be replaced. How do our cells know what to do so perfectly at all times? Of course, this is a great mystery that scientists and theologians have debated passionately. My personal view is that the consciousness of life force pulsates within each one of us, even at the tiniest cellular level. Of course, I can't literally *feel* my cells, but knowing that my body lives in rhythm to this greater life force helps me consciously align my actions and thoughts to this divine wisdom.

We know that our cells must work in harmony with one another to form and maintain the body. Likewise, each one of us is analogous to a single cell pulsating within the universe. When we forget that we are part of this cosmic web, we are in danger of feeling isolated and all alone. This feeling of separation tends to make us go, literally, off beat, which can manifest as physical, psychological, or spiritual ailments.

Just like learning how to swim, living your rhythm at first requires a great deal of concentration, coordination, and practice. If you've been swimming for most of your life, you probably can't remember there was a time before you knew how to swim because it's become so natural to you. But humans aren't fish. We had to start in the shallow end of the pool and learn the kicks, arm strokes, how to float, and how to blow bubbles underwater. To swim, every part of your body must work together in rhythmic coordination. With practice, you eventually learn this new rhythm that allows you to swim in a pool or the Aegean Sea and experience the incredible, buoyant sensation of being one with the water. When you look at rhythm in terms of swimming or even walking, you see how rhythms can give us an incredible amount of freedom.

THE FINE ART OF LISTENING
AND RESPONDING

How do we learn to listen to our inner voice? One way is by making mistakes. The times when we don't listen to ourselves are just as valuable as the times we do. The day after Passover, my client Dalia went to a restaurant for breakfast and ordered pancakes. After eight days of not having any bread products, Dalia wanted to treat herself with this childhood food. When she was young, her mother made pancakes every Saturday, a family ritual that everyone looked forward to. Her inner voice told her that she's sensitive to wheat and that pancakes wasn't what she needed, but she ordered them anyway, with butter and maple syrup just as she had them as a child. After she finished the pancakes, she felt terrible. She was tired, had a headache, and was spaced out the rest of the day.

The only way to get in touch with our inner understanding of how to nourish ourselves is by paying attention—seeing what works and what doesn't work. Not all foods serve us well. If we know a certain food causes a negative reaction (headaches, sore throats, bloated tummy), then we learn to avoid that food. The cleanse is a fantastic opportunity to pay attention to how you feel when you feed yourself clean foods as well as when you add other foods back into your system. Dalia can still eat her pancakes occasionally, for example, but it's with the knowledge that she may suffer the consequences. So be smart about your choices. If you know you have a busy day ahead of you, for which you need to be alert and energetic, then feed yourself foods that fuel you so you can be present for what's needed in your life.

Dalia's mother recently came to visit her in San Francisco. They went out for breakfast and again the menu had pancakes. For a moment, Dalia considered getting them but ultimately decided it wasn't worth it. This time she not only listened, she also *responded*. She ordered the tofu scramble instead.

THE HOLIDAY CYCLE

It's October, and the weather is just beginning to get that chill in the air that lets us know the days are growing steadily darker and colder. On the shelves in the supermarkets, giant-size bags of candy appear in all colors and varieties. It's the beginning of the Halloween season. From corporate offices to hospitals and teachers' lounges, in workplaces across the country bowls of candy and other sweets are put out for everyone's enjoyment. These bowls will steadily be refilled through Halloween, Thanksgiving, Christmas, New Year's, Valentine's Day, and all the way up to Easter. With the warmer weather, the candy bowls will finally disappear. At this point, most of us are so exhausted after six months of perpetual sugar feasting that we're relieved to say good-bye to the sweets. It used to be that feasting only accompanied a time of harvest, celebration, or a successful hunt. Today, we're living most of the year in a feast modality.

The holiday season has its own powerful momentum. Once this sugar and refined carbohydrate train gets started, it's difficult to stop it in its tracks. From candy to pies and other baked goods, holiday foods are everywhere you turn, enticing you to participate in the holiday spirit by having more and more of them. By the time we're making our New Year's resolutions we're just about ready to burst. But the holiday train continues to roll . . . right on through to spring. Unfortunately, too many of us roll right along with it. Or, should I say, we are rolled over by it?

Our natural rhythm in the winter is to slow down, be more quiet, contemplative, and domestic. During the cold winter months, do you feel like staying at home more often? Wanting to take naps on the weekend and just curl up with a good book? If we look at the natural tendency of land animals, we see that they slow down or hibernate during the dark winter months. We also are aligned to these natural seasonal rhythms. Unfortunately, we don't have the luxury to tuck ourselves into our homes for a few months and reemerge when the days grow longer. We have to keep going. One social function of the holidays is to keep us stimulated during this time of year.

One way to make it soundly through the holidays without slipping into the feasting mode is by remaining true to your inner rhythms. Because they usually go overboard during the holidays, two of my clients who are friends decided to support each other by cleansing during Thanksgiving one year. Cleansing gave Sandra and Jackie the structure to remain disciplined during this holiday of plenty. "It was inspirational," they told me. "I didn't feel deprived at all," Sandra marveled. "It was a relief to remove myself from the madness." Even if you don't choose to do a long cleanse during the holidays, you may wish to consider a retreat day after each holiday. For this retreat day, you could feed yourself according to the third phase of the cleanse (see page 143) or just vegetables. These mini-cleanses are a wonderful way to curb the sweet tooth compulsion and maintain balance during the holidays.

YIN AND YANG: LIVING BALANCE

According to Chinese philosophy and medicine, expansion and contraction are the two forces by which the universe maintains its dynamic balance. Also known as yin and yang, this philosophy understands that all life is perpetually in the process of balancing two complementary forces. For every inhalation we take, there's an exhalation. In the morning the sun rises, in the evening it sets. For each and every force in the universe, there exists its complement. In the winter, the trees are bare and dormant. In the summer, they yield new fruit.

Balance is an energetic principle in all natural forms. From the migration of birds to entire ecosystems and the life of a single cell, every aspect of the cosmos is continually in the process of seeking balance. Expansion and contraction represent opposites, but they really are two faces of the same coin. They are neither good nor bad. When a woman experiences a contraction during labor, for instance, her muscles tighten so that the birth canal can expand.

Yin and yang represent a continuum, a full circle. Day may seem to be the antithesis of night, but the rising or setting of the sun doesn't happen all of a sudden. We know that day and night are created by the earth's steady revolution around the sun. Likewise, the yin-yang continuum shows us that all life is in constant motion. When this movement is gentle and responsive, then we experience balance and harmony. You practice subtle responsive movement each time you drive your car. As a new driver, you probably made the common mistake of turning the steering wheel too much, jerking your car all over the road until you got a better feel for the motion. Your mistake was thinking you need big movements of the wheel. In reality you only have to turn the wheel very little, and often, to keep the car evenly between the yellow lines.

Being balanced and calm in the middle of the road isn't the same as living mediocre lives where nothing much happens.

There's a perception that life is more exciting on the edges, whereas balance has no room for passion, thrill, energy, or intensity. The truth is you don't have to be a mountain climber or a surfer riding a twenty-foot wave in Hawaii to experience the thrill of being alive. The same excitement is available to you from within yourself. From the place of internal balance, you can harness your own vibrant and potent life force. This is real excitement, because you aren't dependent on external sources of pleasure for your happiness.

The body's natural inclination is for health, well-being, and vitality, and its natural wisdom is to perpetually strive for balance. It's a beautiful thing. All we have to do is learn to get out of the way! When the body is balanced, our emotions are calm. We aren't prone to great mood swings. We feel equipped to respond to the many surprises that life continually presents us. When the body is at ease, you become like a tranquil pond: Your mind is awake; you have the ability to concentrate; you're open and receptive to your spirit. If our bodies are not in balance, it's as though rocks have been thrown into the pond. The once calm waters become agitated and murky. As long as more rocks aren't thrown into the water, the pond will eventually become placid again.

You will know when your body is balanced. You will feel energetic and physically vibrant, mentally alert and clear, and emotionally open and responsive. The body, mind, and emotions need to be aligned to access the spirit. For the spirit to soar, we need to feed ourselves foods that create lightness of being. Lightness doesn't refer to your weight but to a *feeling* in your body of ease, calm, balance, and open-heartedness. We feel light when we aren't holding on to more than is necessary, when we don't have excess baggage, physically as well as emotionally.

BALANCE MEANS CHANGE

Balance is a dynamic process, not a permanent condition. I can't emphasize this enough. All living organisms are perpetually in a state of change. You aren't the same person you were five years ago or even five minutes ago. So, too, your needs for nourishment continually change. That's because our bodies don't function in a vacuum. Balance is always relative to the person we are today. Who we are in the present moment is influenced by everything that occurs in our lives—how we feel physically, what we ate yesterday, our emotions, age, stress level, physical activities, intellectual demands, travel, time of day, even the weather outside. Nourishment means reestablishing your intimate connection to your body so you know when you are balanced, recognize when you are not, and understand how to respond to your ongoing needs for equilibrium.

One year into a rigorous graduate program, my client Ian realized he needed different foods to help him keep up with all of the hours of studying. After being happy as a vegetarian for many years, his body was informing him that he needed meat. "Meat," he told me in mild disbelief. "I'm eating meat again. I'm studying for exams this week and need a lot of energy. I even had a bison burger last night." When I asked him about his reasons he said, "Eating meat is something I never thought I would do, but I've learned I have to be open to hearing what my body needs."

What happened for Ian beautifully illustrates how our needs for balance change all the time, and how important it is to listen and respond to these changes. For Ian this meant being honest about how he makes decisions about feeding himself. It could have been easy for him to automatically dismiss his internal messages because they signaled him to go against an important aspect of his identity. Instead of getting caught up in his ideas about being a vegetarian, he chose to listen to his body. When he responded to his body's hunger for meat, he learned that this food potently fuels him at this time in his life.

Of course, balance isn't a final destination but an ongoing practice that simply is part of the journey of our lives. Personal and spiritual growth is always ongoing. We just don't end up perfectly realized one day, able to sit back and drink piña coladas for the rest of our lives. No, balance keeps us on our toes and forces us to be aware and responsive. Thankfully, nourishment gives us countless opportunities for balance, the state from which we can directly touch spirit.

BECOMING A SOURCE
OF NOURISHMENT

my monk friend has a weird endearing habit
he weaves sandals and leaves them secretly by the roadside

—IKKYŪ, *fifteenth-century Zen master*

WHEN YOU COME TO THE BRIDGE . . .

There's a story about two men who were friends with a king in a far-off kingdom. One day, the men are caught stealing. The friends are taken to the royal palace, where they admit their culpability before the king. This confession weighs heavily on the king's heart, as the usual punishment for stealing is death. Since the king can't bear to have his friends' blood on his hands, he decides to give them one chance to escape with their lives. "I'll tell you what," says the king. "At the edge of the kingdom is a gorge. I will have a rope strung over its wide mouth. You must walk across that rope. If you reach the other shore safely, then you are free to keep going. Only you must never return to this kingdom."

As they stand at the edge of the gorge, the two men are delighted by their good fortune. How often in life are we given such a second chance? Without a moment's hesitation, the first man safely walks across the rope to freedom. But the second man suddenly feels a touch of vertigo he's never experienced before. He steps up to the edge and pauses, realizing just how narrow the rope is, how deep the chasm, and how far he must cross. His friend motions wildly for him to join him. Standing there at the edge, with certain death behind him and the chance of a new life before him, he shouts: "Tell me, friend, how did you do it? How did you cross?" The other man replies, "I can't tell you exactly. All I know is that when I felt myself lean too much to the left, I leaned to the right."

If the man makes it across, we'll never know. That's where the story ends. One way of looking at life is as a series of bridges to cross. Each bridge represents a new transformation, a new evolution in your spiritual growth as a human being. I believe the point of this parable is to teach us that we always have a choice. Growth perpetually asks us to change. When we come to the major crossing points in our life, we can choose to cross to the other shore—no matter how frightened we are—or we can stay put. You could argue that in this story the men didn't have much choice: They knew they'd be killed if they returned to the kingdom. What kind of choice is that? But they also had the option of attitude. The second man represents our fears, doubts, and unwillingness to let go and trust the unknown. The man who crossed represents our potential to embrace change and step into the unfamiliar. How did he do it? With equanimity, by leaning a little to the left and a little to the right.

Fortunately, very few of us have to walk a narrow rope over dizzying heights to make it to our next stage of evolution—although the way we resist change, we act as though we do have to walk a tightrope. A bridge doesn't have to be dangerous. Bridges can be very solid, and easy to cross. Regardless if you're crossing a rickety old wooden bridge or the Brooklyn Bridge, one thing is true for all of us: Every bridge has its bridge keeper who can help us make the crossing. The first man in the parable advised his friend how to cross. Perhaps you're feeling compelled to nourish yourself in a fuller way as a result of reading this book. If that's the case, then I am a bridge keeper for you right now, just as you've probably helped someone else across in your own way.

The only way to cross from one form of our life to the next is by taking the steps: We can't just talk the talk, we have to walk our walk. Maybe you test the ground a little before you're sure it is solid. Once you know it's okay, you take another step. It takes great courage to act on what you know to be true. If you want to begin gradually by feeding yourself two meals a week that you've cooked from scratch, that's a step. If you do a three-day cleanse, that's also a step. If you decide that it's important to feed yourself and your family organic meats and dairy, that's another step. Usually one step leads to another because each step proves to be beneficial in your life. You don't cross the bridge in a single bound. You do it by starting where you are and taking small steps. And if you need to rest along the way, then you rest.

The beauty of a culture like ours is that you can live your life just about any way you want. When I started to do this work in the 1960s, food and consciousness was relegated to a small subculture. In those days, just being a vegetarian made me unusual. That I was making my own tofu was simply over the top. More than ever, people today are dissatisfied living their lives in tiny little compartments. We are actively looking for ways to integrate all aspects of our lives—physical, spiritual, familial, and vocational—and to nourish ourselves accordingly. It's a lot easier today than it was thirty years ago. Fresh organic vegetables are available all year, and even tofu has become mainstream. Take comfort knowing that you are not alone. Look around you on the bridge and you will see many others who share the same desire for integration, wholeness, and deep meaning in their lives.

Once you've crossed one bridge, you can always visit the place you came from, but you can't live there again. If you grew up eating hamburgers, french fries, and milkshakes, you can have these foods when you're an adult, but only occasionally. Once we experience a deeper level of nourishment, we are more willing to change our patterns. Bridge crossings require us to leave parts of ourselves behind. In this way, each life transformation represents a loss as well as a birth. But you lose only what no longer serves your life's journey. What you gain is what's in your heart of hearts.

In what's become a classic, Bill Moyers and Joseph Campbell discuss the meaning and mystery of life through the lens of mythology in the series *The Power of Myth*. Toward the end of the interview, Campbell makes the startling statement: "I don't believe life has a purpose. Life is a lot of protoplasm with an urge to reproduce and continue in being." Moyers, a bit surprised and indignant, replies: "Not true, not true."

Campbell goes on to explain: "Wait a minute. Just sheer life cannot be said to have a purpose, because look at all the different purposes all over the place. But each incarnation, you might say, has potentiality, and the mission of life is to live that potentiality. How do you do it? My answer is, 'Follow your bliss.' There's something inside you that knows when you're in the center, that knows when you're on the beam or off the beam. And if you get off the beam to earn money, you've lost your life. And if you stay in the center and don't get any money, you still have your bliss." Satisfied with this answer, Moyers now agrees: "I like the idea that it is not destination that counts, it's the journey."

BE A KITCHEN ALCHEMIST

One way to work with transformation on a regular basis is through daily contact with fire. Cooking is an ancient process. Fire is a catalyst for alchemy, and it's an essential element in transforming what comes from the earth into a more digestible form. Most people I work with don't have enough contact with fire, and I think this is true for many people today. With the advent of fast food, convenience foods, microwaves, and supermarket deli sections, we've become a population that doesn't use fire to nourish ourselves. I usually shy away from blanket directives, but I feel so strongly about the missing presence of kitchen fire in our daily lives that I will break my own rule and say: Everyone in this country needs more regular contact with the hearth.

I once had the good fortune to meet a man who worked for the National Park Service in Alaska for many years. When I found out that Ray was an anthropologist who had lived among native Alaskan populations, I couldn't help but ask: "What do they feed themselves?" Some people are intrigued by a culture's political or economic structure. I always want to know what people are eating. After fascinating me with his intriguing tales and observations, Ray was kind enough to lend me an excellent book about the Koyukuk Indian culture, *Tracks in the Wildland*, which he co-authored. In this thorough study I came upon the following passage about the role of fire and food.

"Respect for food is also shown in the way it is eaten. Those who adhere to tradition will not eat outdoors without somehow formalizing the meal—making a fire and perhaps putting down a bed of spruce boughs on which to sit. In past years food was always heated, but today people might just gather around a fire while eating the food cold." Fire is so crucial that one Koyukuk woman warned: "If you don't make a fire, you'll just stay hungry. You might even get sick."

Fire was literally the first spark in human evolution that allowed for all the discoveries and inventions that followed. Embers were guarded day and night because fire was such a precious and difficult element. Today, electricity has taken the place of real fire in most of our homes. Instead of the hearth, our kitchens are stocked with electronic gadgets. Microwaves can warm up frozen dinners in less than five minutes. But don't be fooled. A microwave doesn't create real heat, as does a gas range. Even an electric stovetop is closer to the real fire element.

When you take a meal out of a box or a plastic bag, you have very little involvement with your food. The only creativity that's asked of you is the choice of which box to heat up. Compare that process to cooking, where you have total creativity and freedom to select each ingredient for a meal and then to chop, cut, slice, grate, and mix those ingredients. You are working with all of the elements: earth, air, and water. When you add the element fire to the process, you become an alchemist in your very own kitchen. With the aid of fire, you turn vegetables into soup, raw fish into a sumptuous, edible meal, flour and water into the simple miracle called bread. This transformative, alchemical process is deeply nourishing. On the one hand, we benefit from the literal fruits of our efforts. At the same time, cooking allows us regularly to engage in the act of creation.

At a workshop I once gave, I met a theological student who impressed me with the passion by which she spoke about searching for God in her life. The reason she had come to the workshop was because she wanted to get in touch with, and nourish, deeper parts of herself. During the question and answer period, she asked me a simple question about vegetables. Because she lives alone and cooks mostly for herself, she feeds herself frozen vegetables that she defrosts in the microwave. I noticed that she was wearing very cool colors—blues, whites, and greens. I suggested that she could benefit from using real fire. Even if she ate frozen vegetables, I told her, she should heat them on a gas or electric stove. She was shocked. This was a revolutionary idea. She had never thought that fire could help her connect to her passion and inner development.

I felt a great deal of compassion for this woman. I could see she sincerely wanted to live more vibrantly and yet she was frozen in her life. I felt I had to engage her with something outrageous, so I blurted out, "Wear red underwear!" The words just flew out of my mouth before I could censor myself. After the workshop, she came up to me privately to ask for more information about fire. "Can I put more spice in my food?" she asked. "Absolutely!" I told her to take it another step further and to feed herself more red and yellow vegetables. I could see she was beginning to catch on. When I returned a month later, she again attended the workshop. I noticed her right away. She was dressed in deep cranberry and maroon. The colors looked great on her; they were very warm.

EVERY STAGE OF THE ROSEBUSH

In the year that we worked together, Georgia had made great strides in her self-growth. And then she was diagnosed with cancer for the second time. Georgia's diagnosis hit her very hard. She was upset and angry. For the first time in months, she sat down and ate ice cream—her most addictive food. The next morning Georgia cooked a large pan of greens for herself. As she ate the greens, she said to herself, "This is what I deserve." Yes, she was diagnosed with cancer again. Yes, she was angry. But she realized that she deserves to support herself in a healing and loving way. "So, I'm angry," she told herself. "Does that mean I'm going to hurt myself? I don't deserve that. I deserve this," she thought as she savored another bite of the vibrant greens.

One day soon after, Georgia came to my office for a session. I took her outside into the garden to see the roses, or, rather, to see the rosebush, as the roses had yet to bud. "Every stage of the rosebush," I told her, "is a stage of a beauty." In only a few weeks this thorny plant will develop buds that will burst into fragrant red flowers. I said to her, "Is this bare plant with its potential for growing roses any less beautiful, any less miraculous, than the actual rose?"

Spiritual growth isn't linear. We can't rush it or control it. What we can do is love and nourish ourselves to our utmost capabilities each day. And, perhaps most difficult of all in our culture, we can practice patience. We've grown accustomed to acquiring things quickly and conveniently—information, services, food, material goods. We can learn from the wise counsel Rainer Maria Rilke gives to the young poet, eager to obtain life experience and to become accomplished at his art. "There is no measuring with time, no year matters, and ten years are nothing," Rilke writes. "Being an artist means, not reckoning and counting, but ripening like the tree which does not force its sap and stands confident in the storms of spring without the fear that after them may come no summer. It does come. But it comes only to the patient, who are there as though eternity lay before them, so unconcernedly still and wide. I learn it daily, learn with to which I am grateful: *patience* is everything!"

Georgia and I looked at the rosebush for a little while. "What I'm beginning to realize," she said, "is that I have to be happy with what I've achieved thus far. I have to accept that I'm somewhere on this rosebush and that I have no idea where! I mean, I might be the bud, or the flower that's about to lose its petals. Or I might be part of a cycle like photosynthesis that we don't actually see." She took a deep breath and closed her eyes. When she opened them she said slowly, "I have to learn to be patient with myself, to accept myself with strengths together with my flaws. I have to accept and celebrate myself, regardless of where I am in my life." And then a smile spread across her face. What was left to say? I just beamed back at her.

THE EYE OF THE HEART

Spirit works through the heart, and the language of the heart surpasses the realm of words. Passion, compassion, unconditional love, and the ability to nourish oneself and others are the heart's vernacular. Over the past decades, there has been wonderful and necessary work with mindfulness practice. We have learned from teachers of the East and West how to develop awareness and live all aspects of our lives with greater focus, insight, and equanimity. We learned that no activity is too small or trivial to warrant our mindful attention. Even washing the dishes is an opportunity to practice mindfulness.

What I propose here, however, is a slightly different paradigm to mindful eating and that's heartful nourishment. Nourishment means activating and strengthening the muscles of the heart. It really has very little to do with the mind. Of course a basic intellectual understanding is important. Initially, your intellect must be engaged as you learn the daily practice of nourishment—which foods serve you best, how to prepare them, combine them, when to eat, and so forth. Once you understand the mechanics of nourishment, you take it to the realm of the heart.

The heart is much more than our romantic affections. According to the scholar Abraham Joshua Heschel, the great medieval Jewish thinker Maimonides stated that "the source of our knowledge of God is the inner eye, 'the eye of the heart,' a medieval name for intuition." Our intuition not only is the source of our knowledge of God, but it also is the source of our knowing exactly how to live our lives in each moment. The eye of the heart is the eye of compassion and love by which we recognize ourselves as spiritual beings, beings with a meaning and purpose here on earth. Once we know this to be true in the deepest place in our hearts, then we naturally accept the responsibility to nourish ourselves.

In time, we begin to receive the blessings from regularly drinking this source of nourishment. The more we engage in this authentic place within ourselves, the more present, loving, expressive, dynamic, purposeful, and genuine we become. When we obtain this consciousness, we see that food is just one type of nourishment. All aspects of our lives can nourish us. In turn, we realize, we can be a source of nourishment for others. Like Ikkyū's monk friend, we, too, can help others walk the steps of their journey.

Manifesting and embodying our spirit takes an enormous amount of courage. And it tests us continually. We need to be able to show up for ourselves and have enough heart to say yes no matter how many times we fall down. If we have any inkling of ourselves as spiritual entities, then we have the responsibility to wake up. The more we feed spirit, the more we live spiritual lives. Living a life infused with spirit isn't just about going to a temple, church, mosque, or zendo. It's about how we take care of our children, how we drive the car, talk to our colleagues, and interact with friends, neighbors, store clerks, and strangers. Living a spiritual life happens every day. It's in the details of our lives as well as our attitude. If we are open and willing to receive, then we can see with the eye of our heart and listen to the voice of our intuition. Try this simple exercise. Make a fist. Now open your hand. How did you feel when your hand was in a fist? How about when it was open? Now try the same exercise with your heart.

The healing power of transformational nourishment isn't about never eating sugar again. Healing happens when you are willing to engage in the process of awareness with yourself. As in Georgia's case, healing means being willing to take risks to truly nourish yourself when the easy route would be to disregard or abuse yourself. As most things worthy of our time and attention, nourishment is a process. It's a beginning, not an end. When you commit to a spiritual path, you still have free will. I've been practicing transformational nourishment for most of my life, and I'm still faced with choices each day. I can decide to remain present and loving for myself and others or I can decide to hide under the covers. To be honest, that's not entirely true. You see, the more spirit directs your life, the less willing you are to act in ways that compromise your service to it.

Practice nourishment. Practice it so well, you forget you're even doing it. When we learn something that completely, we have a saying for it. We say that you know it by heart.

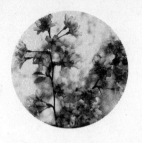

PART FOUR

RECIPES FROM THE HEARTH

Delicious and Simple Meals

That Nourish Body and Spirit

CONTENTS

SOUPS

Baba's Broth (Potassium Broth), 197
Ginger–Leek Miso Soup, 199
Haleakala Red Lentil Soup, 201
Shiitake Mushroom Soup, 202
Silky Asparagus and Celery Soup, 203
Kale and Sweet Potato Soup, 204
Hearty Root Vegetable Soup, 206
Cauliflower Soup, 207

SALADS

Arame Sea Vegetable Salad, 211
Radicchio and Fennel Salad, 212
Watercress Salad, 213
Avocado and Red Onion Salad, 214
Beet and Sorrel Salad, 215
Very Celery Salad, 216
Miso Marinated Onions, 217

DRESSINGS AND SAUCES

Asian Spring Roll Dipping Sauces, 221
Shallot–Herb Dressing, 223
Curried Salad Dressing, 224
Thai Dressing with Basil, 225
Creamy Ginger Vinaigrette, 226
Red Pepper–Avocado Vinaigrette, 227

VEGETABLE DISHES

Cauliflower with Black Sesame Seeds, 231
Braised Cabbage, Fennel, and Leeks, 232
Sauté of Tender Greens, 233
Broccoli Rabe with Pignolia Nuts, 234
Asian Spring Rolls, 235
Cauliflower Curry, 236
Spiced Kale and Escarole, 238
Onions Provençal, 239
Roasted Rutabaga with Beets, 240
Stuffed Dumpling Squash with Hiziki, 241

GRAINS

Sweet Brown Rice with Mushrooms, 245
Quinoa Tabouli, 247
Soba Noodles with Scallions, 248
Crispy Millet, 250
Savory Buckwheat, 251

MAIN DISHES

Ginger Poached Cod with Bok Choy, 255
Spicy Sardine Salad, 256
Salsa Snapper, 257
Tilapia with Sesame–Sea Vegetable Topping, 259
Ceviche, 260
Soul-Satisfying Fish Stew, 262
Lima Bean Dip with Roasted Endive, 263

MAIN DISHES *(continued)*

Festive French Lentils, 265

Black-eyed Peas with Red Onion and Fresh Mint, 266

Simply Spicy Adzuki Beans, 267

Uzbek Chickpeas and Squash, 268

Crispy Sesame Tofu, 269

Golden Tofu Salad with Creamy Ginger Vinaigrette, 270

Satori Tofu, 272

Dijon Grilled Tofu, 273

Josef's Pesto Tofu Bundles, 274

Tofu Spread with Sun-dried Tomatoes and Olives, 275

BREAKFAST

Hash Browns, 279

Rise and Shine Tofu, 280

Irish Oatmeal, 281

Protein Smoothie, 282

FRUIT

Baked Pears with Ginger and Cardamom, 285

Dried Fruit Compote, 286

Applesauce, 287

Summer Fruit with Papaya Sauce, 288

DESSERTS

Almond–Ginger Delights, 291

Sour Cherry–Chocolate Truffles, 292

Hazelnut Macaroons, 293

Poached Figs with Cinnamon and Cloves, 294

Cranberry-Stuffed Pears with Crunch Topping, 295

GLOSSARY OF INGREDIENTS

INTRODUCTION TO RECIPES

The kitchen is my favorite room of the house. I could spend hours in the kitchen. I love the smells, creativity, and coziness. It's no surprise that the kitchen is the place where people most often congregate. In my home, there are always people gathered around our kitchen table, and there's always a pot of something on the stove, from rice to soup and beans. If it's a cold and rainy day, I can go into my pantry with its jars of beans, grains, seeds, and nuts and I'll know that it's a Haleakala Red Lentil Soup day. This simple soup can be made in forty-five minutes, and then it's a source of warmth and nourishment for everyone who comes through the kitchen that day.

The kitchen is the center of transformation in the house. It is one of the only places in our lives where we can regularly engage with fire, the alchemical element that allows us to transform raw ingredients into sumptuous dishes. When I was growing up, my grandmother, my *nene*, was always in the kitchen preparing a meal. The smells of simmering pots constantly permeated the kitchen and wafted through the rest of the house. Rice, chickpeas, pinto beans, lima beans, lamb cooked with cumin, stewed vegetables, beets, tomatoes, green beans, eggplants, fish, olives, feta, goat, and sheep cheeses. The kitchen was a place of incredible activity and the "studio" where I learned about food's endless creative possibilities.

Because I have the good fortune to work at home, I am in and out of the kitchen all day long. In the middle of a client session,

I've been known to jump up and run to my kitchen to give my client a taste of a food that would be beneficial for him or her. Sometimes I'll send clients home with a container of food so they can have it later.

Originally I provided clients with recipes to help them with the cleanse. Over time, I found that people needed a greater variety of ingredients and tastes to sustain this new way of feeding themselves all year long. The recipes here are the culmination of years of experimentation, inspired dishes from my clients, and creative modifications to more traditional recipes. These dishes are delicious, but they won't create an addictive need because the ingredients are so clean. The recipes are free of wheat, refined sugars, and dairy to provide clean, high-energy fuel for most people most of the time.

These recipes are a synthesis of the two culinary styles that have influenced me most, the Japanese and Mediterranean approaches to food. I learned from my native Turkey an appreciation for the freshest fruits and vegetables, good quality olive oil, and simple fish meals. For many years, I have had a deep affinity for Japanese culture, aesthetics, and their sane approach to food. The traditional Japanese diet is primarily based on land vegetables, sea vegetables, rice, and fish, and has impeccable standards for ingredients and aesthetic presentation. In the early 1970s, I was trained by the Japanese master chef Hiroshi Hayashi. Since then, I've traveled to Japan and have hosted many Japanese exchange students in my home, who continued to share with me the simple and elegant aesthetics of their culture, from art to food. You'll notice the influence of both the Mediterranean and Japanese cultures in these recipes.

Most of the recipes are appropriate to use while cleansing. Recipes that have cleanse notes either indicate slight variations to make the recipe cleanse friendly or inform you that the recipe should not be used while you are cleansing. (Desserts are an example of this.)

All of the recipes are relatively quick and easy to prepare. I know people are busy—I'm busy!—so I've developed nourishing recipes that allow you to make a meal from scratch in very little time. To help you decide if you have enough time to make a particular dish, preparation and cooking times are indicated in each recipe. Each recipe also indicates the seasons when fresh produce is available in most temperate climates. This is a guideline only, and it shouldn't prevent you from trying the recipe if you live in a different climate or if the recipe interests you during a different season.

Recipes are written on the page but it's only in your kitchen where they come to life. I invite you to play with these recipes, to make them your own unique creations by modifying the ingredients according to your own needs or culinary flair.

From my hearth to yours, may you be well nourished. Enjoy!

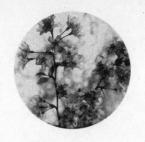

SOUPS

BABA'S BROTH
(POTASSIUM BROTH)

Yield: 8 8-ounce servings
Preparation Time: 10 minutes
Cooking Time: 1½ hours
Seasons: All

Baba is an affectionate term for "father" in many languages, including Turkish, Chinese, and Hindi, and our children have always called their father by this name. Since my husband is the best broth maker in our household, this recipe is named after him. I'm personally fond of a broth made of green vegetables while my husband, who drinks broth all day long, has mastered a heartier broth composed mostly of root vegetables.

Rich in potassium and other minerals, these broths make a very healing drink that's excellent for cleansing or any time of year when you're feeling a bit run down. Drink this broth as a tea throughout the day, or use it as a nourishing stock for other soups.

BABA'S BROTH I

3–4 large kale leaves
1 bunch beet greens
4 stalks celery
1 bunch parsley
8 cups water

Or any of the following:
2 small leeks, rinsed thoroughly,
  roots trimmed, and cut in half
½ bunch scallions
1 bunch watercress
2–3 collard green leaves

BABA'S BROTH II

2 beets
1 celeriac (celery root)
2 burdock roots
1 black radish
1 small rutabaga
1 small purple-top turnip
2 celery stalks
8 cups water

Wash the vegetables and cut the celery, if using, in half. Place all the vegetables into a large soup pot and add the water (the pot should be no more than approximately ¾ full). Bring to a boil. Reduce heat, cover, and simmer for a minimum of 1½ hours. You may keep the pot on the stove for 1–2 days, reheating as desired.

NOTE:

Use the liquid only and discard the vegetables after all the broth has been consumed.

GINGER–LEEK MISO SOUP

Serves 6
Preparation Time: 15 minutes
Cooking Time: 30 minutes
Seasons: All

4 small leeks
1 teaspoon extra-virgin olive oil
2 onions, thinly sliced and cut into
  half-moon strips
2 carrots, matchstick sliced
6 cups water
4 shiitake mushroom caps, thinly sliced
2 ounces firm tofu, cut into
  ½-inch cubes
1 teaspoon freshly grated ginger
½ teaspoon salt
2 tablespoons brown rice miso paste

GARNISH

crumbled wakame sea vegetable
coarsely chopped watercress or arugula leaves

1. Trim the roots off the leeks. Slice off and discard the tough green leaves from the tops of the leeks. Wash the remaining white and light green portions thoroughly in cold water. Make sure to rinse in between the layers, removing any sand. Shake dry and slice thinly.

2. Heat the oil in a large pot and sauté the leeks, onions, and carrots until the vegetables are soft. Add enough water to cover the vegetables and bring to a boil. Add the shiitakes, tofu cubes, grated ginger, and salt. Add more water for a thinner consistency. Reduce heat and simmer, covered, for 25 minutes.

3. In a bowl, dissolve the miso in ½ cup of the hot broth and add to the pot just before serving. Garnish each bowl with wakame and watercress or arugula.

VARIATION:

Replace the tofu with freshly baked white fish, such as haddock, cod, or scrod.

HALEAKALA RED LENTIL SOUP

Serves 4
Preparation Time: 5 minutes
Cooking Time: 45 minutes
Seasons: All

Last winter my family vacationed in a cottage 3,000 feet up on Mt. Haleakala, a beautiful volcanic mountain in Maui. One evening we had a bonfire for our friends. The cool mountain weather called for food that would warm us all up. I was inspired to re-create a lentil soup I had tasted in a Tibetan restaurant in Boston. Everyone was wild about this soup and asked for the recipe. From Tibet to Boston to Maui to your kitchen, may you be equally nourished and inspired to add your own touch to this simple, satisfying soup.

1 cup red lentils
4 cups water
½ cup mild salsa, chunky style, or ½ cup chopped tomatoes
1 small onion, finely chopped
¼ teaspoon cinnamon
½–1 teaspoon cumin
¼ teaspoon coriander
½ teaspoon salt

GARNISH

sprig of fresh mint or coarsely chopped cilantro

Place lentils, water, salsa, and onion in a medium soup pot. Bring to a boil over medium-high heat. Reduce heat, cover, and simmer for 15 minutes or until lentils are soft. Stir in cinnamon, cumin, coriander, and salt. Simmer for another 20–30 minutes. Garnish individual bowls with fresh mint or cilantro just before serving.

SHIITAKE MUSHROOM SOUP

Serves 4
Preparation Time: 10 minutes
Cooking Time: 10–12 minutes
Seasons: Spring/Summer

1 tablespoon extra-virgin olive oil
1 small onion, finely chopped
10 fresh shiitake mushroom caps, sliced
½ teaspoon salt
4 cups boiling water
1–2 tablespoons freshly squeezed lime juice
1½ teaspoons crumbled wakame, dulse, or kelp sea vegetable
freshly ground black pepper to taste

GARNISH

1 cup arugula or bok choy, coarsely chopped
1 finely chopped scallion

1. In a medium soup pot, heat olive oil over medium heat. Add the onion, mushroom caps, and salt, and sauté for about 5 minutes or until the onion is soft.

2. Add the boiling water to the onion and mushrooms and cook for 5 more minutes. Turn off the heat and season with lime juice, sea vegetable, and pepper, adjusting as necessary. Garnish individual bowls with arugula or bok choy and scallions just before serving.

SILKY ASPARAGUS AND CELERY SOUP

Serves 6–8
Preparation Time: 15 minutes
Cooking Time: 30 minutes
Seasons: Spring/Fall

4 small leeks
1 tablespoon extra-virgin olive oil
1½ pounds asparagus, finely chopped
1 pound celery, finely chopped
6 cups water or vegetable stock
1 teaspoon ground coriander
1 teaspoon ground cumin
1 teaspoon salt
½ teaspoon freshly ground black pepper

GARNISH

1 bunch watercress, leaves and stems coarsely chopped

1. Trim the roots off the leeks. Slice off and discard the tough green leaves from the tops of the leeks. Wash the remaining white and light green portions thoroughly in cold water. Make sure to rinse in between the layers, removing any sand. Shake dry, then slice them thinly on the diagonal.

2. Heat the oil in a large soup pot over medium-high heat. Add the leeks and sauté for 3–5 minutes until they just begin to soften. Add the asparagus and celery and sauté for 5–8 more minutes.

3. Add the water or stock and seasonings and bring to a boil. Cover, reduce heat, and simmer for 15 minutes until all the vegetables are soft. Puree in a blender and season with salt and pepper to taste. Garnish individual bowls with the watercress just before serving.

KALE AND SWEET POTATO SOUP

Serves 6–8
Preparation Time: 25 minutes
Cooking Time: 50 minutes
Seasons: Fall/Winter

1 head garlic
3 tablespoons extra-virgin olive oil
4 small leeks
1 sprig fresh rosemary
4 sweet potatoes, peeled and
   cut in ½-inch pieces
6 cups water or vegetable stock
1 small bunch kale, fibrous stems removed,
   leaves chopped
1 teaspoon salt
½ teaspoon freshly ground black pepper

1. Preheat the oven to 300°. Slice off the top of the garlic head, exposing the cloves slightly. Place the garlic in a small shallow baking dish. Drizzle 1 tablespoon of oil over the top of the exposed cloves, cover, and bake for 20–25 minutes. Remove from the oven and let cool, squeeze the cloves out of their papery shells, and set aside.

2. Trim the roots off the leeks. Slice off and discard the tough green leaves from the tops of the leeks. Wash the remaining white and light green portions thoroughly in cold water. Make sure to rinse in between the layers, removing any sand. Shake dry, then slice them thinly on the diagonal.

3. Heat 2 tablespoons of oil in a large soup pot. Sauté the leeks, rosemary sprig, and roasted garlic cloves over medium heat. Cook until the leeks become translucent. Add the sweet potatoes and continue cooking, stirring frequently, until the potatoes begin to soften, about 10 minutes.

4. Add the water or stock. Bring to a low boil, cooking until the potatoes are tender, about 12 minutes. Add more liquid if a thinner consistency is

desired. Add the kale, cooking just until it begins to wilt, about 4 minutes. Season with salt and pepper.

VARIATION:

For a creamy consistency, puree some or all of the soup in a blender before adding the kale.

HEARTY ROOT VEGETABLE SOUP

Serves 6
Preparation Time: 20 minutes
Cooking Time: 1 hour
Seasons: Fall/Winter

2 tablespoons extra-virgin olive oil
2 medium onions, diced
2 stalks celery, chopped
6 cloves garlic, peeled and minced
1–2 carrots, peeled and chopped
2–3 small potatoes, peeled and chopped
1 small fennel bulb, quartered, cored, and chopped
1 small rutabaga (yellow turnip), peeled and chopped
6 cups water
1 tablespoon miso paste, brown rice or mellow white
1 small bunch parsley or cilantro, chopped

GARNISH

⅓ cup thinly sliced scallions or 1 bunch watercress, leaves and stems
coarsely chopped

1. Heat the oil in a large soup pot over medium heat. Sauté the onions, celery, and garlic for 3–5 minutes, stirring frequently. Add the carrots, potatoes, fennel, and rutabaga. Add the water, making sure there is enough to generously cover the vegetables. Cover the pot and bring to a boil. Reduce the heat and simmer for 45–60 minutes.

2. In a bowl, dissolve the miso paste in ½ cup of the hot soup broth.

3. Turn the heat off and stir in the dissolved miso and chopped parsley or cilantro. Garnish with scallions or watercress before serving.

Variation:

For a creamy consistency, puree some or all of the soup in a blender.

CAULIFLOWER SOUP

Serves 6
Preparation Time: 25 minutes
Cooking Time: 40 minutes
Seasons: Fall/Winter

2 tablespoons extra-virgin olive oil
1 small onion, coarsely chopped
3 cloves garlic, peeled and minced
1 teaspoon ground cumin
½ teaspoon ground coriander
1 teaspoon salt
½ teaspoon freshly ground black pepper
1 large head cauliflower, chopped
4–6 carrots, chopped
5 cups water or vegetable stock

GARNISH

nori granules

1. In a large soup pot, heat the oil over medium heat. Add the onion and garlic and sauté until they're lightly browned. Add the spices, salt, and pepper and stir constantly for 1 minute. Add the cauliflower and carrots, stirring to combine with the onion and spices.

2. Add the water or stock, making sure there is enough liquid to cover the vegetables. Bring to a boil, then cover, and reduce heat to medium-low. Simmer until the vegetables are soft.

3. Puree the soup in batches in a blender. Garnish individual bowls with nori granules just before serving.

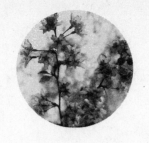

SALADS

ARAME SEA VEGETABLE SALAD

Serves 6
Preparation Time: 30 minutes
Seasons: All

This delicate sea vegetable has a milder taste than other seaweeds. For this reason, arame is a wonderful way to enter the realm of sea vegetables if you've never had them before. From the most conservative eaters who are squeamish about even the words "sea vegetables" to fussy teenagers, everyone I serve this dish instantly loves it. The trick to this exquisite salad is making sure that you use plenty of toasted sesame oil.

1 package (1.76-oz) dried arame sea vegetable
1–2 red bell peppers, seeded and chopped
6 scallions, diagonally sliced
3 tablespoons unrefined toasted sesame oil
2 tablespoons brown rice vinegar
1 tablespoon tamari or 2 tablespoons Bragg
1 tablespoon gomasio (sesame salt)

1. Soak the arame for 20 minutes in a medium-size bowl with just enough cold water to cover.

2. Drain the liquid from the arame and place the arame into a serving bowl. Add the remaining ingredients and toss gently. The salad keeps well refrigerated for a few days.

CLEANSE NOTE:

Substitute brown rice vinegar with 2 tablespoons freshly squeezed lime juice.

RADICCHIO AND FENNEL SALAD

Serves 4
Preparation Time: 20 minutes
Seasons: All

1 small fennel bulb, quartered, cored, and thinly sliced
½ head of radicchio, halved, cored, and thinly sliced
½ cup carrots, matchstick sliced

DRESSING

2 limes, juiced
1 teaspoon honey (optional)
grated zest of 1 orange
½ teaspoon salt
½ teaspoon freshly ground black pepper
¼ cup extra-virgin olive oil

1. Combine the fennel, radicchio, and carrots in a serving bowl.

2. In a small bowl, mix together the lime juice, honey, orange zest, salt, and pepper. Whisk in the oil. Add the dressing to the salad and toss well.

WATERCRESS SALAD

Serves 2–4
Preparation Time: 15 minutes
Seasons: All

2–3 bunches watercress, leaves and stems chopped
1 red bell pepper, seeded and thinly sliced
¼ cup grated daikon radish
¼ cup sunflower sprouts
¼ cup mung bean sprouts
½ teaspoon dulse granules
2 teaspoons extra-virgin olive oil
¼ teaspoon salt
1 lime, juiced

Combine all the ingredients and toss gently.

WATERCRESS VARIATION 1:

In a bowl, mix together 1 cup grated black radish and 1 cup grated yellow turnip. Stir in juice from 1 lemon and mix well. Serve over a bed of chopped watercress.

WATERCRESS VARIATION 2:

In a bowl, mix together 1 cup grated daikon radish and 1 cup grated carrot. Stir in ½ cup sunflower sprouts and juice from 1 lemon. Serve over a bed of chopped watercress.

AVOCADO AND RED ONION SALAD

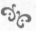

Serves 4–6
Preparation Time: 20 minutes
Seasons: Spring/Summer/Fall

2 ripe avocados, sliced into ½ inch cubes
½ medium red onion, very thinly sliced
    and cut into half-moon strips
1 jalapeño, seeded and minced (optional)
1 lemon
salt and freshly ground black pepper to taste
dulse and kelp granules
fresh mixed greens

1. In a large bowl, mix together the avocado, red onion, and jalapeño.

2. Peel off the rind of the lemon with a vegetable peeler or knife, avoiding the white pith, and slice it into julienne strips. Slice the lemon in half and then juice it.

3. Gently mix the lemon rind, lemon juice, salt, and black pepper with the avocado and onion. Sprinkle with dulse and kelp granules. Serve over a bed of fresh greens.

NOTE:

Jalapeño peppers are very hot and need to be handled with care. Wear rubber gloves to protect your hands from burns when seeding and mincing the peppers.

BEET AND SORREL SALAD

Serves 4–6
Preparation Time: 20 minutes
Marinating Time: 10 minutes
Seasons: Spring/Summer/Fall

3–4 small raw beets, scrubbed
3 lemons, juiced
freshly ground black pepper
1 medium bunch sorrel, chopped

Grate the beets by hand or in a food processor. Mix the beets, lemon juice, and black pepper together. Marinate for at least 10 minutes. Serve over the sorrel.

NOTE:

Sorrel can be substituted with arugula or watercress.

VERY CELERY SALAD

Serves 4
Preparation Time: 10 minutes
Marinating Time: 30 minutes
Seasons: Fall/Winter

In my view, celery is one of the most underappreciated vegetables today. This salad boldly brings celery to center stage, and the combination of tangy seasonings really brings out its subtle flavor. Celery is fantastic for people who love crunchy food. This quick recipe also expands our concept of salad from the standard leafy green mixture to other vegetables.

2 tablespoons extra-virgin olive oil
1½ tablespoons fresh lemon juice
2 cloves garlic, peeled and minced
½ teaspoon salt
½ teaspoon freshly ground black pepper
1 teaspoon celery seeds
6 stalks celery, thinly sliced on the diagonal
3 scallions, thinly sliced on the diagonal

1. Mix together the oil, lemon juice, garlic, salt, pepper, and celery seeds in a small bowl. Set aside.

2. In a large bowl, combine the celery and scallions. Add the dressing and mix thoroughly. Cover and refrigerate for about 30 minutes to allow the celery to marinate in the dressing. This salad is delicious alone or served over a bed of arugula or other salad greens. It also makes a great topping for steamed fish.

MISO MARINATED ONIONS

Serves 6
Preparation Time: 30 minutes
Cooking Time: 5 minutes
Seasons: Fall/Winter

2 large sweet onions, very thinly sliced
    and cut into half-moon strips
1 shallot, thinly sliced
boiling water
¼-inch piece ginger root, julienned

DRESSING

⅓ cup sake
⅓ cup mirin
2 tablespoons tamari or Bragg
3 tablespoons raw cane sugar
⅓ cup mellow miso paste

1. Place the onions and shallot in a heat-proof bowl and cover them with boiling water. Soak for 10 minutes, and then drain the water.

2. Meanwhile, heat the sake, mirin, tamari, and sugar in a small pot. Bring just to boiling and turn off the heat. Stir the miso into the hot liquid until it is dissolved. Let cool. Pour the dressing over the onions and mix in the ginger slices. Cool the onions in the refrigerator before serving. This dish lasts up to a week in the refrigerator, with the onions getting more tender and flavorful the longer they marinate.

CLEANSE NOTE:

This recipe is not appropriate for the cleanse.

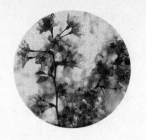

DRESSINGS AND SAUCES

ASIAN SPRING ROLL DIPPING SAUCES

Yield: ¼ cup
Preparation Time: 10 minutes
Seasons: All

These lively dressings are fantastic dipping sauces for the Asian Spring Rolls (see page 235). They're also great for green salads, steamed vegetables, or to dress up canned tuna or salmon.

MISO WASABI SAUCE

1 tablespoon light or mellow miso
3 tablespoons water
¼ teaspoon wasabi mustard
1 tablespoon chopped scallions

Combine all ingredients in a small bowl. Mix well until the mixture is smooth. Add more water for a thinner consistency.

CLEANSE NOTE:

This recipe is not appropriate for the cleanse.

SPICY GINGER MISO SAUCE

1 teaspoon light or mellow miso
3 tablespoons sesame oil
2 tablespoons freshly squeezed lemon juice
¼ teaspoon wasabi mustard
½ teaspoon freshly grated ginger
pinch of crushed red pepper

Combine all ingredients in a small bowl. Mix well until the mixture is smooth.

CLEANSE NOTE:

This recipe is not appropriate for the cleanse.

FRESH HERB SAUCE

3 tablespoons extra-virgin olive oil or flax seed oil
2–3 tablespoons freshly squeezed lemon juice
½ cup loosely packed mint leaves
½ cup loosely packed basil leaves
¼ teaspoon salt

Blend all ingredients quickly in a blender or food processor.

VARIATION:

Substitute 3 chopped scallions and ½ cup cilantro in place of the
mint and basil leaves.

SHALLOT–HERB DRESSING

Yield: 1 cup
Preparation Time: 15 minutes
Seasons: All

This tangy dressing makes use of fresh and dried herbs. Feel free to substitute any of them with your own preferred combinations.

> 2 tablespoons extra-virgin olive oil
> 1 shallot, peeled and minced
> 1 lemon, juiced
> ½ lime, juiced
> handful of minced fresh parsley
> ½ teaspoon dried basil
> ½ teaspoon dried oregano
> ½ teaspoon dried dill
> 1 clove garlic, peeled and minced
> ¼ teaspoon salt
> ¼ teaspoon freshly ground black pepper
> vegetable broth or water to dilute

Mix all ingredients together in a glass jar. Seal tightly and shake well. For a more even consistency, puree together in a blender or food processor.

CURRIED SALAD DRESSING

Yield: 1/3 cup
Preparation Time: 5 minutes
Seasons: All

¼ cup extra-virgin olive oil
2 tablespoons rice wine vinegar
1 teaspoon Dijon mustard
1 teaspoon tamari or Bragg
¼ teaspoon ground cumin
½ teaspoon curry powder
salt and black pepper to taste

Combine all ingredients in a small bowl or a jar that has a tight-fitting lid. Whisk or shake the closed jar well.

VARIATION:

They say variety is the spice of life. To spice up this Indian-inspired dressing, try adding any or all of the following: chopped roasted almonds, unrefined toasted sesame oil, chopped scallions, or finely diced shallots.

CLEANSE NOTE:

This recipe is not appropriate for the cleanse.

THAI DRESSING WITH BASIL

Yield: ¾ cup
Preparation Time: 15 minutes
Seasons: All

This dressing is equally tasty on salads as it is with fish or tofu. It's also good for an Asian-style coleslaw made with shredded cabbage, grated carrots, and chopped scallions.

2 tablespoons extra-virgin olive oil
2½ tablespoons freshly squeezed lemon juice
¼ teaspoon salt
¼ cup vegetable broth or water
1 teaspoon dulse granules or Bragg (optional)
1 clove garlic, peeled and minced
½ jalapeño pepper, seeded and diced (optional)
2 scallions, thinly sliced
8 mint leaves, finely chopped
2 tablespoons chopped basil
2 tablespoons chopped cilantro or parsley

In a medium bowl, whisk together all ingredients.

NOTE:

Jalapeño peppers are very hot and need to be handled with care. Wear rubber gloves to protect your hands from burns when seeding and mincing the peppers.

CREAMY GINGER VINAIGRETTE

Yield: ⅔ cup
Preparation Time: 10 minutes
Seasons: All

¼ cup unrefined toasted sesame oil
2 tablespoons rice vinegar
4 ounces silken tofu
1 tablespoon freshly grated ginger
1 teaspoon honey or maple syrup
2 teaspoons tamari or Bragg

Combine all ingredients in a blender or food processor. Blend or pulse just until creamy.

CLEANSE NOTE:

This recipe is not appropriate for the cleanse.

RED PEPPER–AVOCADO VINAIGRETTE

Yield: 1 cup
Preparation Time: 15 minutes
Seasons: Summer/Fall

1 red bell pepper, seeded and chopped
½ ripe avocado
4 cloves garlic, peeled and minced
1 lemon or lime, juiced
freshly ground black pepper to taste
water

Cut the avocado in half, remove the pit, and scoop out the flesh with a spoon. Place the avocado and the other ingredients in a blender or food processor. Blend or pulse until creamy. For a thinner dressing, mix in a tablespoon of water at a time until you reach the desired consistency.

VARIATION:

Add 3–5 fresh basil leaves, 1 teaspoon of dulse or kelp granules, or 2–3 scallions.

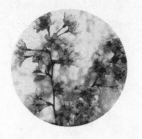

VEGETABLE DISHES

CAULIFLOWER WITH BLACK SESAME SEEDS

Serves 4
Preparation Time: 10 minutes
Cooking Time: 30 minutes
Seasons: All

1 head cauliflower, cut into large florets
2 tablespoons unrefined toasted sesame oil
½ teaspoon salt
¼ teaspoon freshly ground black pepper
1 tablespoon black sesame seeds

1. Preheat the oven to 400°. Place the cauliflower florets into a baking dish. Add the oil, salt, and pepper, and mix well to coat evenly. Bake uncovered for 20–30 minutes, until the cauliflower feels tender when punctured with a fork.

2. While the cauliflower is roasting, place the sesame seeds in a dry cast iron or heavy skillet over medium heat. Cook, stirring continuously, until they begin to pop and smell fragrant, about 3 minutes. Remove from the heat and set aside.

3. Remove the cauliflower from the oven and transfer to a serving dish. Sprinkle with the toasted sesame seeds and serve.

SUMMER VERSION:

Lightly steam the cauliflower until it's tender but still firm. Dress with the juice of 1 lemon or lime, 2 tablespoons sesame oil, and top with black sesame seeds.

BRAISED CABBAGE, FENNEL, AND LEEKS

Serves 4–6
Preparation Time: 20 minutes
Cooking Time: 30 minutes
Seasons: Spring/Fall

2–3 small leeks
2 tablespoons extra-virgin olive oil
4 cloves garlic, peeled and minced
½ teaspoon salt
1 small head of napa cabbage, thinly sliced
1 small fennel bulb, thinly sliced
½ cup vegetable stock or water
½ lemon, juiced

1. Trim the roots off the leeks. Slice off and discard the tough green leaves from the tops of the leeks. Wash the remaining white and light green portions thoroughly in cold water. Make sure to rinse in between the layers, removing any sand. Shake dry, then slice into thin rings.

2. Heat the oil in a large skillet over medium heat. Sauté the garlic for 30 seconds. Add the leeks and salt and continue sautéing for 2–3 minutes, stirring frequently.

3. Stir in the cabbage, fennel, vegetable stock or water, and lemon juice. Turn the heat to medium-high and continue cooking for 3–5 minutes. Reduce the heat and simmer, uncovered, stirring occasionally, until most of the liquid evaporates, about 25 minutes.

VARIATION:

For a more colorful dish, substitute red cabbage for the napa cabbage.

SAUTÉ OF TENDER GREENS

Serves 4–6
Preparation Time: 15 minutes
Cooking Time: 10 minutes
Seasons: Spring/Summer/Fall

This dish of cool-weather greens and warming spices strikes the perfect harmony. For a real work of art, serve the vegetables on a green platter or bowl.

> 2 small leeks
> 1 teaspoon extra-virgin olive oil
> 1 bunch asparagus, chopped into 2-inch pieces
> 2 bunches watercress, leaves and stems coarsely chopped
> ½ teaspoon ground coriander
> ½ teaspoon ground cumin
> salt and pepper to taste

1. Trim the roots off the leeks. Slice off and discard the tough green leaves from the tops of the leeks. Wash the remaining white and light green portions thoroughly in cold water. Make sure to rinse in between the layers, removing any sand. Shake dry, then slice them thinly crosswise.

2. In a large skillet, heat the oil over medium heat. Sauté the leeks for 3 minutes or until they begin to soften. Add the asparagus and cook for another 5–8 minutes, until tender but still crisp. Add the watercress, coriander, cumin, salt, and pepper and stir constantly for another 30–60 seconds. Turn off the heat and adjust seasonings to taste.

BROCCOLI RABE WITH PIGNOLIA NUTS

Serves 4
Preparation Time: 15 minutes
Cooking Time: 10 minutes
Seasons: Spring/Summer/Fall

*1 bunch broccoli rabe, stems and florets
chopped to 1½-inch lengths
1 red bell pepper, seeded and thinly sliced to
1½-inch-long strips
1 tablespoon pignolia nuts
juice of 1 lime
2 teaspoons extra-virgin olive oil
1 teaspoon tamari or Bragg
2 cloves garlic, peeled and minced
½ teaspoon freshly ground black pepper
¼ teaspoon crushed red pepper*

1. Set a steamer basket in a large pot with a small amount of water. Bring the water to a boil, reduce the heat, and place the broccoli rabe and red pepper into the steamer. Cover and steam for about 3–5 minutes, just until the broccoli rabe begins to turn bright green. Immediately place the vegetables in a serving dish.

2. In a dry cast iron or heavy skillet, cook the pignolia nuts over medium-high heat, stirring regularly until they turn light brown, about 3 minutes. Set aside.

3. Mix together the lime juice, oil, tamari, garlic, and seasonings in a small bowl. Add the dressing to the vegetables and toss well. Garnish with the toasted pignolia nuts.

CLEANSE NOTE:
Substitute the pignolia nuts with chopped roasted walnuts or
almonds.

ASIAN SPRING ROLLS

Yield: 1 roll
Suggested Serving: 3 rolls per person
Preparation Time: 10 minutes
Seasons: Spring/Summer/Fall

1 large (8-inch) spring roll rice wrapper (see note)
½ sheet of nori sea vegetable
1 arugula leaf, or 2 sprigs watercress
small amount of sprouts (sunflower, radish, broccoli, etc.)
2½-inch piece of scallion
4–5 fresh mint leaves
2–3 thin slices of ripe avocado

1. Place the rice wrapper under hot water from your kitchen sink until pliable, about 5–10 seconds. Remove immediately. Gently shake off any excess water and set onto a dry, flat surface.

2. Place the half sheet of nori on the bottom part of the rice wrapper (the part nearest you). Add the remaining ingredients on top of the nori, starting with the arugula and sprouts, leaving a 1-inch space around the edges. Be careful not to overstuff the roll, as the wrapper will tear if it is too full.

3. Start rolling from the bottom, folding in the sides as you roll. The rice wrapper is sticky when it's wet, so it will adhere to itself. The rolls are best served the same day. If storing in the refrigerator, cover them well with plastic wrap or a damp cloth so that they don't dry out.

VARIATION:

Try filling the roll with feta cheese, vermicelli, or any combination
of fresh vegetables and herbs that are in season.

NOTE:

Rice wrappers are available at Asian markets or whole foods stores.

CAULIFLOWER CURRY

Serves 4–6
Preparation Time: 20 minutes
Cooking Time: 25 minutes
Seasons: Fall/Winter/Spring

When I'm in Maui I buy my vegetables from Nui twice a week. She grows a variety of vegetables in her garden in Kula, especially greens—lettuces, Oriental vegetables, scallions, basil, mint, arugula, and unusual local greens and squashes. I love supporting her small business, and would ask her about vegetables that I had never tried before. One day I picked up a head of cauliflower from her, which inspired me to make this curry dish. Nui's cauliflower is the most tender and flavorful cauliflower I have ever tasted.

2 tablespoons extra-virgin olive oil
1 onion, chopped
4–6 cloves garlic, peeled and minced
1 small head of cauliflower, cut into large florets
3 small potatoes, chopped
¾ cup salsa, or 3 fresh chopped tomatoes
½ cup water
½ cup fresh or frozen broad beans, string beans, or snap peas, cut into 1-inch pieces
1 teaspoon curry powder
½ teaspoon ground cumin
¼ teaspoon ground cinnamon
½ teaspoon salt

In a large skillet, heat the oil over medium heat. Sauté the onion and garlic until the onion is soft, about 5–8 minutes. Add the cauliflower, potatoes, salsa, and water. Cover and simmer for about 20 minutes, until the potatoes are soft. Stir in the beans or peas and remaining seasonings, and cook, covered, for 5 more minutes, until the flavors are blended.

VARIATION:

Add tofu while cooking the cauliflower and potatoes to create a hearty, one-skillet meal.

SPICED KALE AND ESCAROLE

Serves 6
Preparation Time: 15 minutes
Cooking Time: 10 minutes
Seasons: Fall/Winter

These lovely greens were served at a luncheon after a group of women helped me prepare my garden for the winter. After a few hours in the crisp autumn weather, we all needed to warm up. The aroma of the cooking spices filled the kitchen, drawing everyone around the stovetop. Not only was the fragrance wonderful, but the spices actually created heat in the body and left everyone feeling warm and satisfied.

2 tablespoons extra-virgin olive oil
1 teaspoon freshly grated ginger
2 teaspoons ground cumin
2 teaspoons ground turmeric
1 teaspoon ground coriander
½ teaspoon salt
½ teaspoon freshly ground black pepper
1 bunch kale, fibrous stems removed, leaves coarsely chopped
1 bunch escarole, coarsely chopped

GARNISH

1 bunch scallions, diagonally sliced

1. Combine the oil, ginger, and spices together in a cup and mix well. Heat a large skillet over medium heat for 1 minute. Add the oil and spice mixture and cook for 30 seconds or until the spices are fragrant. If the mixture becomes too pasty, add a few drops of water to thin out.

2. Add the kale, stirring well to coat the leaves with the oil and spices. Cook for 3–5 minutes, stirring once. Mix in the escarole and cook for another 3–4 minutes. The greens should be vibrant in color and tender but not wilted. Garnish with fresh scallions before serving.

ONIONS PROVENÇAL

Serves 4
Preparation Time: 10 minutes
Cooking Time: 45 minutes
Seasons: Fall/Winter

I am a real onion lover. Onions, scallions, leeks, garlic, chives, you name it. I love them cooked, baked, or raw. When I cook, I'm always interested in working with vegetables to bring forth the fullest flavor while not sacrificing the potency of their nutrients. Roasting on high heat with oil and a few savory herbs creates a buttery rich, sweet and savory vegetable side dish.

6 medium yellow onions, quartered
2 teaspoons salt
2 tablespoons extra-virgin olive oil
2 tablespoons dried herbal mixture of thyme,
    rosemary, tarragon, and basil

Preheat the oven to 400°. Combine all ingredients in a large glass casserole dish and mix well. Cover tightly and bake for 45 minutes.

VARIATION:

Replace the dried herbs with crushed red pepper and black pepper.

ROASTED RUTABAGA WITH BEETS

Serves 6
Preparation Time: 15 minutes
Cooking Time: 60 minutes
Seasons: Fall/Winter

Roasted root vegetables have become my fall and winter mainstay. There's nothing like the earthiness of roasted root vegetables to ground your energy and keep you warm on cold blustery days. I've discovered that the key to consistently delicious vegetables is roasting on very high heat with enough high-quality olive oil to coat all the vegetables.

1 large rutabaga (yellow turnip), cut into 2-inch chunks
3 medium beets, quartered
4–6 onions, quartered
2–3 tablespoons extra-virgin olive oil
1 teaspoon salt
½ teaspoon freshly ground pepper
dulse granules
juice of ½ lemon

Preheat the oven to 450°. Arrange the vegetables in a casserole dish (a glass Pyrex dish works well). Add the oil, salt, and pepper and mix well. Cook for 45–60 minutes, stirring occasionally for even roasting. Remove from the oven and sprinkle with dulse granules and lemon juice.

VARIATION:

Just about any kind of root vegetable is delicious roasted. In addition to rutabagas and beets, try roasting any combination of carrots, parsnips, sweet potatoes, purple potatoes, and white potatoes. The tubers also can be cut into long, thick shoestring shapes for variety.

STUFFED DUMPLING SQUASH WITH HIZIKI

Serves 4–6
Preparation Time: 20 minutes
Cooking Time: 50 minutes
Seasons: Fall/Winter

3 dumpling squashes, halved and seeded
2 tablespoons extra-virgin olive oil
dulse granules or ¼ teaspoon salt
1 package (1¾-oz.) hiziki sea vegetable
2 medium onions, thinly sliced
1 red bell pepper, seeded and sliced
5 shiitake mushroom caps, sliced
2 teaspoons unrefined toasted sesame oil

1. Preheat the oven to 450°. Brush the inside of the squash halves with 1 tablespoon of the oil and sprinkle with dulse granules. Bake the squash halves in a shallow baking dish, cavity side up, for 30 minutes. Remove from oven.

2. While the squash is baking, prepare the hiziki stuffing. Place the hiziki in a large bowl and fill the bowl with enough cold water to cover the sea vegetable. Soak for 10 minutes, drain, and set aside.

3. In a large skillet heat 1 tablespoon of oil over medium-high heat and sauté the onions, red pepper, and shiitakes for 5 minutes. Stir in the drained hiziki and continue sautéing for another 10 minutes. Remove from the heat and drizzle with sesame oil. Fill each squash with the hiziki stuffing and serve immediately.

NOTE:

If you cannot find dumpling squash, acorn and buttercup squashes are equally delicious.

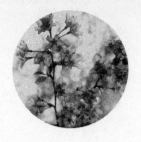

GRAINS

SWEET BROWN RICE WITH MUSHROOMS

Serves 4
Preparation Time: 15 minutes
Cooking Time: 55 minutes
Seasons: All

1 cup uncooked short grain
sweet brown rice
2 cups water
1 tablespoon extra-virgin olive oil
4 cloves garlic, peeled and minced
½–1 tablespoon minced ginger
1 cup assorted mushroom caps (shiitake, cremini,
porcini, etc.), thinly sliced
2–3 tablespoons mirin
¼ cup minced scallions
½ cup frozen sweet green peas
1–2 tablespoons tamari or Bragg
¼ cup vegetable stock
¼ teaspoon freshly ground black pepper

1. To cook the rice, place 1 cup uncooked rice in a pot with 2 cups of water. Bring to a boil, uncovered. Reduce the heat to medium-low, cover, and cook for about 40 minutes, or until all the water is absorbed. Turn off the heat and let stand, covered, for 5 minutes before using.

2. In a large skillet, heat the oil over medium-high heat. Sauté the garlic, ginger, and mushrooms for 2 minutes. Reduce the heat to medium and add the mirin. Cover and cook for 3–4 minutes. Add the scallions and cook, covered, for an additional 2 minutes.

3. Stir in the rice and peas and cook, uncovered, for 2–3 minutes. Add the tamari, vegetable stock, and pepper. Cook, stirring, until the liquid is almost all absorbed.

VARIATION:

If using dried mushrooms, save the soaking liquid to use in place of the vegetable stock.

CLEANSE NOTE:

Use shiitake mushrooms only and substitute the mirin with 2–3 tablespoons of freshly squeezed lemon or lime juice.

QUINOA TABOULI

Serves 4
Preparation Time: 30 minutes
Cooking Time: 25 minutes
Marinating Time: 30 minutes
Seasons: Summer/Fall

1 cup quinoa, rinsed
2 cups water
1 bay leaf
2 cloves garlic, peeled and minced
⅔ cup chopped scallions
1 cup tomatoes, seeded and chopped (optional)
⅔ cup seeded and chopped cucumbers
2½ tablespoons chopped fresh mint,
*   or 1½ tablespoons dried mint*
1 cup finely chopped parsley
3 tablespoons freshly squeezed lemon juice
salt and freshly ground black pepper to taste
1 bunch sorrel, chopped

1. Place the quinoa, water, and bay leaf in a medium pot. Bring to a boil, cover, and simmer on low for 20 minutes, or until all the water is absorbed. Let the quinoa cool to room temperature, then transfer to a serving bowl and discard the bay leaf.

2. Mix together the garlic and scallions with the quinoa. Stir in the remaining chopped vegetables and herbs. Add the lemon juice, salt, and pepper, and toss well. Adjust the seasonings as necessary. Set aside for at least 30 minutes before serving, which will give the flavors time to blend together. Fluff with a fork and serve on a bed of sorrel.

VARIATION:

Replace the tomatoes with 1 small grated beet.

SOBA NOODLES WITH SCALLIONS

Serves 6
Preparation Time: 10 minutes
Cooking Time: 10 minutes
Seasons: Spring/Summer

Soba noodles are a traditional Japanese staple, and are frequently used in soups. Made from buckwheat, soba has a nutty flavor and is more nourishing than wheat pasta. Served at room temperature, this is a great summer pasta dish that can be made in large quantities for a festive meal with friends.

1 pound soba (buckwheat) noodles, cooked
*   according to directions on package*
3 tablespoons unrefined toasted sesame oil
3 tablespoons rice vinegar
2 cloves garlic, peeled and minced
½ teaspoon freshly grated ginger
½ teaspoon crushed red pepper
*   (optional)*
2 tablespoons tamari or Bragg
1 bunch scallions, thinly sliced

GARNISH

2 sheets nori, cut into strips
1 tablespoon gomasio (sesame salt)

Place the cooked noodles in a serving bowl. Mix in the oil, vinegar, seasonings, and scallions and toss. Garnish with the nori strips and gomasio. Serve at room temperature.

VARIATION:

Udon noodles can be used in place of soba noodles.

CLEANSE NOTE:

This recipe is not appropriate for the cleanse.

CRISPY MILLET

Serves 2–3
Preparation Time: 10 minutes
Cooking Time: 30 minutes
Seasons: Fall/Winter

½ cup millet
1½ cups boiling water
olive oil spray
salt and freshly ground black pepper

1. Over a medium-high flame, heat a large cast iron or oven-proof skillet. Place the millet into the skillet and pour in the boiling water. Turn the heat to medium-low and cover. Cook for about 20 minutes, or until all the water is absorbed.

2. Place an oven rack on the topmost rung of the oven. Preheat the oven to broil.

3. Remove the millet from the heat and spray (or brush) oil evenly over the cooked millet. Place the skillet into the oven and broil for 6–8 minutes, until golden brown and crispy. Remove from the oven and season with salt and pepper. Serve as a side dish in place of rice or other grains.

VARIATION:

To enhance the nutty flavor of millet, roast the millet in a dry skillet until it becomes golden brown and fragrant before adding the boiling water.

SAVORY BUCKWHEAT

Serves 4–6
Preparation Time: 5 minutes
Cooking Time: 40 minutes
Seasons: Fall/Winter

This humble grain is often overlooked today. Once upon a time, buckwheat, also known as kasha, was a staple of our "Old Country" ancestors from Europe and Russia. Buckwheat also makes an excellent stuffing for winter squashes, such as acorn, dumpling, and spaghetti squash. Follow the recipe for savory buckwheat, then fill half a baked squash with the grain. Brush with olive oil and bake for another 5 minutes, or until the buckwheat gets crispy on top.

2 teaspoons extra-virgin olive oil
2 medium onions, thinly sliced
1 cup buckwheat (kasha)
¼ teaspoon salt
2 cups boiling vegetable stock or water
1 teaspoon thyme
1 teaspoon sage
¼ teaspoon freshly ground black pepper

Heat the oil in a pot over medium-high heat. Add the onions and sauté for 5 to 7 minutes, stirring frequently. Add the buckwheat and salt, and continue to stir. Pour in the boiling vegetable stock or water. Reduce the heat and simmer, uncovered, for about 30 minutes, just until most of the liquid is absorbed. Turn off the heat. When the grains are soft, mix in the herbs and black pepper.

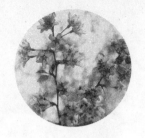

MAIN DISHES

GINGER POACHED COD WITH BOK CHOY

Serves 4
Preparation Time: 15–20 minutes
Cooking Time: 10–15 minutes
Seasons: All

1 cup water
2 cloves garlic, peeled and sliced
1½-inch-long piece fresh ginger, julienned
(about 1 heaping tablespoon)
2 tablespoons tamari or Bragg
3 scallions, diagonally sliced
¼ cup freshly squeezed lemon juice
2 pounds cod fillets (of even thickness), rinsed
1 pound bok choy, stalks and leaves quartered
(approximately 4-inch-long pieces)

GARNISH

thin lemon slices
chopped parsley

1. In a deep skillet, bring the water, garlic, ginger, tamari, scallions, and lemon juice to a boil. Place the cod fillets into the skillet and lower the heat to medium. Cover the skillet and poach for 7–10 minutes, until the fish starts to become opaque.

2. Scatter the bok choy evenly over the fish, cover, and cook an additional 1–2 minutes. Bok choy cooks very quickly. When the leaves turn bright green, turn off the heat and uncover the skillet. Garnish with lemon slices and parsley. Serve hot.

SPICY SARDINE SALAD

Serves 2
Preparation Time: 10 minutes
Cooking Time: 10 minutes
Seasons: All

People often turn up their noses at sardines. But sardines are a power-packed potent food—an excellent source of protein, calcium, and essential fatty acids. Canned sardines are readily available, easy to travel with, and require no cooking. If you've been mixing the same tuna fish salad for years, then try spicing things up with this delicious recipe.

> 2 tablespoons extra-virgin olive oil
> 1 large red onion, thinly sliced and
>   cut into half-moon strips
> pinch of salt
> 1 teaspoon ground cumin
> 1 teaspoon ground coriander
> pinch of chili powder
> 7½ ounces (2 cans) water-packed sardines,
>   drained
> juice of 1 lemon
> 1 bunch arugula or watercress, coarsely chopped

Heat the oil in a skillet over medium-high heat. Add the onion and sauté with a pinch of salt. After 2 minutes, mix in the cumin, coriander, and chili powder. Continue sautéing, stirring frequently, until the onion is tender and translucent, about 5 more minutes. Transfer from the skillet to a serving bowl and let cool. Add the sardines and lemon juice and mix well. Serve over a bed of fresh arugula or watercress.

VARIATION:

Instead of sardines, use 1 can wild Alaskan salmon.

SALSA SNAPPER

Serves 4
Preparation Time: 15 minutes
Marinating Time: 30 minutes
Cooking Time: 10 minutes
Seasons: All

½ cup *freshly squeezed lime juice*
½ teaspoon *ground cumin*
½ small *jalapeño, seeded and minced*
   (optional)
½ teaspoon *salt*
½ teaspoon *freshly ground black pepper*
2 pounds (4 fillets) *snapper or other firm white fish*
   like tilapia or orange roughy, rinsed
1 tablespoon *extra-virgin olive oil*
1 jar (16-oz.) *tomato salsa, or 2 cups*
   chopped fresh tomatoes

GARNISH

1 small bunch *fresh parsley, cilantro, or scallions,*
   finely chopped
lime wedges

1. Whisk together the lime juice, cumin, jalapeño, salt, and pepper in a small bowl. Place the fish fillets into a large, deep dish and cover them with the lime juice marinade. Marinate the fish for at least 30 minutes, turning each fillet over once while marinating.

2. Heat the oil in a large skillet over medium heat. Add the fish fillets, remaining marinade, and salsa to the skillet. Cover and simmer for 8–10 minutes, until the salsa starts to boil and the meat of the fish becomes opaque.

3. Transfer the fish and salsa to a serving platter. Garnish with the chopped fresh herbs and lime wedges. Serve hot.

NOTES:

Fresh salsa can be used instead of store purchased. To make your own salsa, combine 3 chopped large tomatoes, 1 diced small red onion, and 1 finely chopped bunch cilantro. Mix with ¼ cup freshly squeezed lime juice, 3 cloves garlic (minced), salt, and black pepper to taste.

Jalapeño peppers are very hot and need to be handled with care. Wear rubber gloves to protect your hands from burns when seeding and mincing the peppers.

TILAPIA WITH SESAME– SEA VEGETABLE TOPPING

Serves 4
Preparation Time: 20 minutes
Cooking Time: 15 minutes
Seasons: All

¼ cup sesame seeds
¼ cup crumbled wakame sea vegetable
3 cloves garlic, peeled and minced
3 tablespoons chopped parsley
2 pounds tilapia fillets (or other white fish such as cod,
     sole, or flounder), rinsed
freshly ground black pepper
1 tablespoon unrefined toasted sesame oil
juice of 1 lemon
¼ cup vegetable stock

1. Toast the sesame seeds in a dry skillet over medium heat. Cook them, stirring continuously, until golden brown and fragrant, about 3–5 minutes. Combine the toasted sesame seeds and wakame in a spice grinder or blender and pulse until a coarse powder is formed. Place the sesame–wakame mixture into a bowl and mix thoroughly with the minced garlic and chopped parsley. (A suribachi or mortar and pestle also do the trick nicely.)

2. Preheat the oven to 400°. Prepare the fish fillets by sprinkling each side with black pepper. Place in a baking dish and cover with the sesame–sea vegetable topping.

3. In a separate bowl, mix together the sesame oil, lemon juice, and vegetable stock. Pour the liquid into the bottom of the baking dish. Bake, uncovered, for about 12–15 minutes or until the fish flakes.

CEVICHE

Serves 2
Preparation Time: 45 minutes
Marinating Time: 5 hours
Seasons: Spring/Summer

This dish is inspired by traditional Peruvian and Ecuadoran cuisine. Citrus juices not only flavor the fish, they also "cook" it through the long, double marinating process.

1 pound uncooked cod (or any lean white fish),
rinsed and cut into 1½-inch chunks

MARINADE 1

⅓ cup freshly squeezed lime juice
⅓ cup freshly squeezed lemon juice
½ teaspoon whole oregano leaves
2 bay leaves

MARINADE 2

1 tablespoon extra-virgin olive oil
⅓ cup freshly squeezed lemon juice
⅓ cup freshly squeezed lime juice
¼ teaspoon pepper
¼ teaspoon ground cumin
½ teaspoon fresh thyme leaves
1 medium tomato, finely chopped
½ medium red onion, finely chopped
1 fresh jalapeño pepper, seeded and minced (optional)
1 tablespoon finely chopped fresh cilantro or parsley

1. Place the fish in a large non-reactive bowl (glass or ceramic works well) and cover it entirely with the lime and lemon juice. Add the oregano and bay

leaves. Cover and marinate for 4 hours (or up to overnight) in the refrigerator. You will know the fish has "cooked" when it looks whitish-opaque. Remove it from the refrigerator, drain the juice, and discard the bay leaves.

2. Combine all the ingredients for the second marinade in a medium bowl. Add the marinade to the drained fish and mix well. Cover and refrigerate for 1 more hour. Serve chilled over a bed of mixed greens. Ceviche keeps well in the refrigerator for up to 2 days.

NOTE:

Jalapeño peppers are very hot and need to be handled with care. Wear rubber gloves to protect your hands from burns when seeding and mincing the peppers.

SOUL-SATISFYING FISH STEW

Serves 4
Preparation Time: 20 minutes
Cooking Time: 30–40 minutes
Seasons: Fall/Winter/Spring

2–3 small leeks
2 tablespoons extra-virgin olive oil
2 teaspoons freshly grated ginger
2–3 carrots, matchstick sliced
6 shiitake mushroom caps, sliced
2–3 large potatoes, cut in ½-inch cubes
2 tablespoons tamari or Bragg
1 tablespoon wakame or dulse granules
1 pound white fish fillets: haddock, sole, cod, or tilapia, rinsed
4 stalks bok choy, chopped
3 tablespoons arrowroot (optional)

GARNISH

4 scallions or a handful of arugula, chopped

1. Trim the roots off the leeks. Slice off and discard the tough green leaves from the tops of the leeks. Wash the remaining white and light green portions thoroughly in cold water. Make sure to rinse in between the layers, removing any sand. Shake dry and slice thinly.

2. In a large soup pot, heat the oil over medium heat. Sauté the leeks and ginger for 2–3 minutes. Add the carrots, shiitakes, potatoes, tamari, wakame or dulse, and enough water to cover the vegetables. Bring to a boil, reduce heat, and simmer, covered, for 15 minutes.

3. Add the fish fillets and simmer, covered, for another 10–15 minutes. Mix in the bok choy.

4. Dissolve the arrowroot in 3 tablespoons cold water. Add to the stew and stir for 1 minute until the stew thickens. Remove from the heat and garnish individual bowls with scallions or arugula. Serve immediately.

LIMA BEAN DIP WITH
ROASTED ENDIVE

Serves 4–6
Preparation Time: 15 minutes
Cooking Time: 20 minutes
Seasons: Spring/Summer

16 ounces fresh or frozen lima beans (or fava beans)
1 teaspoon extra-virgin olive oil
3 cloves garlic, peeled and minced
1 large onion, finely chopped
½ cup freshly squeezed lemon juice
⅓ cup vegetable stock
dash of coriander
½ teaspoon salt
1 head Belgian endive

1. If using fresh beans, peel and discard the outer shells. If using frozen beans, defrost them before starting. In a medium pot, bring water to a boil and add the beans. Blanch the beans for 3–4 minutes, strain, and set aside.

2. Heat the oil in a deep skillet over medium heat and sauté the garlic and onion. Add the beans and sauté for 10–12 minutes until tender. Stir in most of the lemon juice (you will need some for the endive), vegetable stock, coriander, and salt, and cook for 2 minutes.

3. Puree the bean mixture in a blender or food processor until the mixture becomes smooth. Place the bean dip in a bowl.

4. For the endive: Preheat the oven to broil. Peel apart the leaves of the endive and spread them on a cookie sheet. Lightly brush each leaf with oil and just a drop or two of lemon juice. Broil for about 1 minute. The endive must be checked constantly to avoid burning. Spread the lima bean dip on each endive leaf and serve slightly warm or at room temperature. This dip will keep for a few days stored in a sealed container in the refrigerator.

NOTE:

Instead of using a blender or food processor, you can mash the beans
with the back of a spoon or fork, which produces a heartier
consistency for the dip.

FESTIVE FRENCH LENTILS

Serves 6
Preparation Time: 15 minutes
Cooking Time: 45 minutes
Seasons: Spring/Summer/Fall

4 cups water
1 cup French green lentils, picked through for stones and rinsed
1 small bunch flat-leaf parsley, finely chopped
6 scallions, finely chopped
1 sweet red pepper, chopped
1 yellow pepper, chopped
3 tablespoons unrefined toasted sesame oil
3 tablespoons brown rice vinegar
juice of 1 lemon or lime
2 tablespoons tamari or Bragg
½ teaspoon crushed red pepper
1 teaspoon salt
½ teaspoon fresh ground black pepper

Bring the water and lentils to a boil in a medium pot. Reduce the heat, cover, and simmer for 45 minutes. Drain the water and transfer the lentils to a serving bowl. Let cool. Combine with the vegetables, seasonings, and spices and toss gently. Serve at room temperature.

VARIATION:

Roast the peppers instead of using them raw.

CLEANSE NOTE:

Substitute the brown rice vinegar with extra lemon or lime juice.

BLACK-EYED PEAS WITH RED ONION AND FRESH MINT

Serves 4
Preparation Time: 10 minutes
Season: Summer

2 cups cooked or canned black-eyed peas, drained
1 small red onion, thinly sliced into rings
2 cloves garlic, peeled and minced
4 stalks celery, finely chopped
⅓ cup freshly squeezed lemon juice
3 tablespoons extra-virgin olive oil
½ teaspoon salt
½ teaspoon freshly ground black pepper
1 cup coarsely chopped fresh mint

In a large serving bowl, combine all the ingredients except for the mint. Mix well. Stir in the chopped mint just before serving. Serve at room temperature.

SIMPLY SPICY ADZUKI BEANS

Serves 2–3
Preparation Time: 10 minutes
Cooking Time: 20 minutes
Seasons: Fall/Winter/Spring

2 tablespoons extra-virgin olive oil
1 small onion, diced
2 cloves garlic, peeled and minced
1 jalapeño pepper, seeded and minced
2 cups cooked or canned adzuki beans
¼ cup liquid from the can or water
1 teaspoon ground cumin
½ teaspoon salt
pinch of freshly ground black pepper

GARNISH

1–2 tablespoons chopped scallions

In a large skillet, heat the oil over medium heat. Sauté the onion for 5–7 minutes until browned. Add the garlic and jalapeño and continue sautéing for another 5 minutes, stirring frequently. Stir in the beans, liquid, and seasonings and cook, covered, for 10 minutes over medium-low heat, stirring occasionally. Garnish with scallions before serving.

NOTE:

Jalapeño peppers are very hot and need to be handled with care. Wear rubber gloves to protect your hands from burns when seeding and mincing the peppers.

UZBEK CHICKPEAS AND SQUASH

Serves 6
Preparation Time: 10 minutes
Cooking Time: 30–40 minutes
Seasons: Fall/Winter

1 tablespoon extra-virgin olive oil
2 small onions, chopped
1 cup butternut squash, coarsely chopped
2 teaspoons ground cumin
½ teaspoon ground coriander
½ teaspoon paprika
½ cup chopped fresh tomatoes, or chunky tomato sauce or salsa
1 cup canned chickpeas with ½ cup liquid, or 1 cup cooked
*   chickpeas with ½ cup cooking liquid*
½ teaspoon salt

In a large pot, heat the oil over medium heat and sauté the onions for 3–5 minutes. Add the squash and sauté for 5 more minutes. Stir in the spices and tomatoes. Add the chickpeas with the ½ cup liquid. Cover and simmer for 30–40 minutes. Season with salt. Serve hot as a main meal.

CRISPY SESAME TOFU

Serves 4
Preparation Time: 15 minutes
Marinating Time: 1 hour
Cooking Time: 25 minutes
Seasons: All

3 tablespoons extra-virgin olive oil
3 tablespoons tamari or Bragg
3 tablespoons freshly grated ginger
6–8 cloves garlic, peeled and minced
½ teaspoon crushed red pepper or to taste
1 pound extra-firm tofu, pressed to remove excess water,
*   sliced ½-inch thick*
2–3 tablespoons unhulled sesame seeds

1. Combine the oil, tamari, ginger, garlic, and crushed red pepper in a small bowl and mix well.

2. Arrange the tofu slices in a single layer in a baking dish and add the marinade. Let the tofu marinate for an hour in the refrigerator, turning each piece over at least once.

3. Preheat the oven to 400°. Sprinkle the tofu with sesame seeds. Bake, uncovered, for 25 minutes, or longer for crispier tofu.

GOLDEN TOFU SALAD WITH CREAMY GINGER VINAIGRETTE

Serves 4
Preparation Time: 25 minutes
Marinating Time: 30 minutes
Cooking Time: 15 minutes
Seasons: All

1 tablespoon extra-virgin olive oil
1 pound extra-firm tofu, pressed to remove
   excess water, cut in ½-inch cubes
2 carrots, grated
2 scallions, diagonally sliced
2 tablespoons chopped parsley

VINAIGRETTE

¼ cup unrefined toasted sesame oil
2 tablespoons rice vinegar
4 ounces silken tofu
1 tablespoon freshly grated ginger
1 teaspoon honey or maple syrup
2 teaspoons tamari or Bragg

GARNISH

1 tablespoon gomasio (sesame salt)

1. In a large, heavy skillet, heat the oil over medium heat. Add the tofu and brown well on all sides, about 12–15 minutes. Remove from heat to a large bowl and let cool. Combine the carrots, scallions, and parsley with the tofu and mix well.

2. Place all the vinaigrette ingredients into a blender or food processor. Blend or pulse until creamy.

3. Add the dressing to the tofu salad and blend gently but thoroughly. Cover and refrigerate for at least 30 minutes. Serve cold over a bed of greens, garnished with gomasio before serving.

VARIATION:

Substitute the carrots and the scallions with 1 cup finely chopped fresh kale and 2 tablespoons finely chopped fresh fennel greens.

CLEANSE NOTE:

This recipe is not appropriate for the cleanse.

SATORI TOFU

Serves 4
Preparation Time: 15 minutes
Cooking Time: 35 minutes
Seasons: All

3 tablespoons extra-virgin olive oil
1 pound extra-firm tofu, pressed to remove
   excess water, cut in ½-inch cubes
2 medium onions, finely chopped
2 stalks celery, finely chopped
2 cloves garlic, peeled and minced
1 tablespoon freshly grated ginger
½ cup salsa or chopped fresh tomatoes
2 tablespoons tamari or Bragg
2 tablespoons brown rice vinegar
1 cup water

1. In a large, heavy skillet, heat 2 tablespoons of oil and arrange the tofu in one layer. Cook over medium heat until the tofu is golden on all sides, about 12–15 minutes. Place the tofu in a bowl and set aside.

2. In the same skillet, heat 1 tablespoon of oil and cook the onions, celery, and garlic over medium heat for 5 minutes, stirring occasionally. Meanwhile, in a small bowl mix together the ginger, salsa, tamari, brown rice vinegar, and water.

3. Add the cooked tofu to the skillet and stir in the sauce mixture. Simmer, uncovered, until the sauce is reduced by half, about 15 minutes. This dish is excellent served hot or at room temperature, and is just exquisite the next day. Keep stored in refrigerator for up to a few days.

CLEANSE NOTE:

Substitute the brown rice vinegar with 2 tablespoons lemon juice.

DIJON GRILLED TOFU

Serves 4
Preparation Time: 10 minutes
Marinating Time: 1 hour
Cooking Time: 15–20 minutes
Seasons: All

½ cup freshly squeezed lemon juice
¼ cup Dijon mustard
2 tablespoons tamari or Bragg
⅓ cup extra-virgin olive oil
3–4 teaspoons freshly grated ginger
3–6 cloves garlic, peeled and minced
½ teaspoon salt
½ teaspoon freshly ground black pepper
1 pound extra-firm tofu, pressed to remove
   excess water, cut into 1-inch slices

GARNISH

2 scallions, finely sliced

1. In a large bowl, combine the lemon juice, mustard, tamari, oil, ginger, garlic, salt, and pepper and mix well. Add the tofu to the bowl with the marinade. Cover and let stand in the refrigerator for at least 1 hour, turning each piece of tofu at least once during this time.

2. Remove the tofu from the refrigerator and drain the excess marinade, retaining it for later. Place the tofu on a fish grilling screen and grill for 5–7 minutes per side. Alternatively, place the tofu in a baking dish, cover with half the marinade, and broil in a preheated oven for 20–25 minutes.

3. Heat the remaining marinade in a saucepan and pour it over the tofu before serving. Garnish with the scallions.

CLEANSE NOTE:

This recipe is not appropriate for the cleanse.

JOSEF'S PESTO TOFU BUNDLES

Serves 4
Preparation Time: 30 minutes
Cooking Time: 15 minutes
Seasons: Summer/Fall

2 tablespoons extra-virgin olive oil
1 pound extra-firm tofu, pressed to remove excess water,
  cut into ½-inch-thick rectangles
2 teaspoons tamari or Bragg
dulse granules

PESTO

4 cups fresh basil leaves
½ cup extra-virgin olive oil
¼ cup organic almonds
6–8 cloves garlic, peeled
¼ teaspoon salt

1 tomato, sliced
nori sheets, cut into ½-inch strips

1. In a large, heavy skillet, heat the 2 tablespoons of oil and arrange the tofu in one layer. Cook over medium heat until the tofu is golden on all sides, about 12–15 minutes. Season with tamari and dulse granules. Remove from heat and cool to room temperature.

2. Place all the pesto ingredients into a blender or food processor and blend or pulse until the mixture forms into a paste.

3. Assemble each bundle in the following order: tofu, tomato, 1 teaspoon of pesto. Wrap the strip of nori around the center of the bundle and seal the ends together by moistening one edge with water.

VARIATION:

Replace the pesto with a few fresh basil leaves.

TOFU SPREAD WITH SUN-DRIED TOMATOES AND OLIVES

Serves 4–6
Preparation Time: 15 minutes
Seasons: Summer/Fall

1 pound firm tofu, crumbled
¼ cup sun-dried tomatoes, soaked in hot water and drained
½ cup pitted black olives, rinsed in water
¼ cup capers, rinsed in water
3 cloves garlic, peeled and minced
¼ cup chopped flat-leaf parsley
3 tablespoons freshly squeezed lemon juice
¼ cup extra-virgin olive oil
freshly ground black pepper to taste

Place all ingredients in a blender or food processor. Blend or pulse until well combined and creamy. Use as a spread on rice cakes, as a sandwich filling, or as a dip with vegetables.

CLEANSE NOTE:

This recipe is not appropriate for the cleanse.

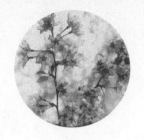

BREAKFAST

HASH BROWNS

Serves 6
Preparation Time: 10 minutes
Cooking Time: 20 minutes
Seasons: Fall/Winter/Spring

3 tablespoons extra-virgin olive oil
2 medium onions, chopped
1 teaspoon salt
4 medium potatoes with skins, baked, cooled, and chopped
1 teaspoon paprika
½ teaspoon freshly ground black pepper

1. In a large, heavy skillet, heat 1 tablespoon of oil over medium-high heat. Add the onions and ½ teaspoon salt and sauté for 5–7 minutes until the onions are lightly browned.

2. Add the potatoes with the remaining ½ teaspoon of salt, 2 table-spoons of oil, paprika, and black pepper. Cook for about 15 minutes, turning the mixture occasionally, until the potatoes are well browned.

VARIATIONS:

Add chopped almonds and chopped cilantro or parsley while cooking.
Use 2 white potatoes and 2 sweet potatoes.

NOTE:

Bake the potatoes the night before for quick and easy breakfast preparation.

RISE AND SHINE TOFU

Serves 2–4
Preparation Time: 15 minutes
Cooking Time: 20 minutes
Seasons: All

This bright and colorful tofu dish is a spicy way to start your day. Because this tofu dish is so versatile, it invites a little adventure into your kitchen. Try using diced scallions, finely chopped broccoli, cilantro, collard greens, or shredded nori in place of any of the vegetables listed below. For an even spicier jump start to your morning, add hot sauce or salsa just before serving.

> *2 tablespoons extra-virgin olive oil*
> *1 large onion, finely chopped*
> *½ teaspoon salt*
> *½ teaspoon turmeric*
> *½ teaspoon coriander*
> *¼–½ teaspoon cayenne, depending on desired spiciness*
> *1 pound extra-firm tofu, drained and cut into 1-inch cubes*
> *1 small red bell pepper, seeded and diced*
> *1 small orange or yellow pepper, seeded and diced*
> *¼ pound shiitake or crimini mushrooms, thinly sliced*
> *1 medium bunch kale, fibrous stems removed, leaves finely chopped*

1. In a large skillet, heat the oil over medium heat and sauté the onion, salt, and spices until the onion turns brown, about 5 minutes.

2. Stir in the tofu, peppers, and mushrooms and continue sautéing for another 7–10 minutes, stirring frequently.

3. Add the kale on top of the vegetables and tofu and cover the skillet. Cook for 2 more minutes, stir well, and serve hot.

IRISH OATMEAL

Serves 2–3
Preparation Time: 5 minutes
Cooking Time: 40 minutes
Seasons: Fall/Winter/Spring

2 cups water
½ cup Irish steel-cut oats
½ teaspoon ground cinnamon
¼ teaspoon ground cloves
¼ teaspoon ground cardamom
2 tablespoons coarsely chopped walnuts

Bring the water to a boil in a pot set over medium-high heat. Stir in the oats. When the oats begin to thicken, reduce the heat to low, cover, and simmer for 40 minutes, stirring occasionally. Remove from the heat and stir in the spices and walnuts. Serve hot.

VARIATION:

Mix in almond, oat, or soy milk or a dollop of yogurt before serving.

CLEANSE NOTE:

This recipe is not appropriate for the cleanse.

PROTEIN SMOOTHIE

Serves 1
Preparation Time: 10 minutes
Seasons: Spring/Summer/Fall

½ *banana*
½ *cup frozen or fresh berries—strawberries,*
   blueberries, raspberries, or blackberries
1 cup almond, rice, or soy milk
1 scoop protein powder

Place all the ingredients into a blender, or use an immersion blender, and blend until smooth. Add more milk or water for a thinner consistency.

CLEANSE NOTE:

This recipe is not appropriate for the cleanse.

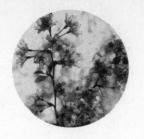

FRUIT

BAKED PEARS WITH GINGER AND CARDAMOM

Serves 2
Preparation Time: 10 minutes
Cooking Time: 20 minutes
Seasons: Fall/Winter

3 ripe pears, cored and quartered
1 tablespoon freshly grated ginger
1 teaspoon ground cardamom
1 tablespoon currants
water

Preheat the oven to 350°. Place the pears in an ovenproof dish and coat them with the ginger, cardamom, and currants. Add enough water to cover the bottom of the dish. Cover and bake for 30–40 minutes, or until the pears are soft. Serve as a breakfast dish or dessert.

VARIATION:

Replace the pears with apples and the currants with fresh cranberries or dried cherries.

DRIED FRUIT COMPOTE

Serves 4
Preparation Time: 10 minutes
Cooking Time: 15–20 minutes
Seasons: Fall/Winter

1 cup any combination of dried fruit (prunes,
  apples, apricots, pears, peaches), rinsed
¼ cup currants, rinsed
1 cinnamon stick
½ teaspoon almond extract
4 slices of fresh ginger (1 tablespoon)
rind of ½ lemon, cut into strips
water
juice of 1 lemon or lime

1. In a small pot, combine the dried fruit, currants, cinnamon stick, almond extract, ginger, and lemon rind strips. Fill the pot with enough water to cover the fruit by 2 inches. Bring to a boil. Reduce heat and simmer, covered, for 5–10 minutes. Add the lemon or lime juice and simmer, covered, for another 10 minutes.

2. Remove from heat when the fruit becomes plump and tender, but not mushy. Discard the cinnamon stick, ginger, and lemon rind before serving.

CLEANSE NOTE:

Eliminate the almond extract.

APPLESAUCE

Serves 4
Preparation Time: 15 minutes
Cooking Time: 20 minutes
Seasons: Fall/Winter/Spring

12 apples, cored, peeled, and chopped
⅓ cup water
1–2 tablespoons freshly squeezed lemon juice
pinch of salt
1 tablespoon cinnamon

Place all the ingredients into a large pot. Mix well and bring to a boil. Reduce the heat, cover, and simmer for 20 minutes, until the apples are soft. Cook longer if you want a smoother sauce. For a creamy treat, serve with rice, almond, or soy milk (except when cleansing).

VARIATIONS:

Use 4 peeled and chopped pears in place of 4 of the apples.
Add ½–¾ cup fresh cranberries to the last 5 minutes of cooking.

NOTE:

Any mix of the softer varieties of apples works well, especially Cortland, Empire, and McIntosh.

SUMMER FRUIT WITH PAPAYA SAUCE

Serves 6
Preparation Time: 25 minutes
Season: Summer

1 vanilla bean or 1 teaspoon vanilla extract
2 small ripe papayas, peeled, pitted, and coarsely chopped
1 cup fresh nectarines, sliced
1 cup fresh apricots, sliced
1 cup fresh papaya, sliced
1 cup blueberries, rinsed and drained
1 cup banana, sliced
2 plums, thinly sliced

GARNISH

fresh mint

1. Cut the vanilla bean in half lengthwise, and scrape out the seeds with the back of knife. Place the vanilla bean seeds or vanilla extract and chopped papaya in a blender. Puree until smooth, adding a small amount of water to achieve a thinner consistency, if desired. Set aside.

2. Wash, cut, and combine the fruit in a large bowl and mix together. Divide the fruit salad into individual servings and drizzle with the papaya sauce. Garnish with sprigs of fresh mint.

VARIATIONS:

You can make apricot sauce instead of papaya sauce by using 6–8 pitted fresh apricots.
For an alternative fruit salad, try 1 cup fresh chopped peaches, 2 sliced kiwis, 1 cup chopped pears, 1 cup halved strawberries, 1 cup chopped bananas, and 2 chopped plums.

CLEANSE NOTE:

Eliminate the vanilla extract.

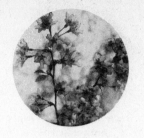

DESSERTS

ALMOND–GINGER DELIGHTS

Yield: 24 confections
Preparation Time: 25 minutes
Seasons: All

These confections evolved out of the Cranberry-Stuffed Pears recipe (page 295). They were made in a pinch when I wanted to make a quick dessert but there wasn't enough time to bake the pears. I just took the "crunch topping" idea and assembled it in a slightly new way. The end result is a delicious treat that's deceptively simple to make.

1 cup roasted unsalted almonds
½ cup crystallized ginger
2 tablespoons maple syrup
1 teaspoon cocoa powder, plus extra for coating

Place all ingredients in a blender or food processor. Blend or pulse until the almonds are finely ground and everything is well combined to form a sticky mass. Form into ½-inch balls. If desired, roll the balls in cocoa and shake off the excess. Stores well in the refrigerator.

CLEANSE NOTE:

This recipe is not appropriate for the cleanse.

SOUR CHERRY–CHOCOLATE TRUFFLES

Yield: 24 truffles
Preparation Time: 20 minutes
Seasons: All

½ cup roasted almonds
6 squares bittersweet chocolate (70 percent cocoa)
1 cup dried sour cherries
¼ cup maple syrup
3 tablespoons cocoa powder
1 tablespoon vanilla

1. To roast the almonds, preheat the oven to 350°. Spread the nuts in one layer on an ungreased baking pan. Bake for 7–10 minutes, until lightly browned. Remove from the oven and let the almonds cool. Grind them in a blender or food processor. Place on a large plate and set aside.

2. Melt the chocolate in a double boiler. Place all the ingredients, except the almonds, into a blender or food processor. Blend or pulse until it forms a well-blended sticky mass, about 3 minutes. Form into ½-inch balls.

3. Roll each truffle in the ground almonds, covering them completely with the nuts. Store in an airtight container in the refrigerator or freezer.

VARIATION:

Dust the truffles with cocoa powder instead of ground almonds.

CLEANSE NOTE:

This recipe is not appropriate for the cleanse.

HAZELNUT MACAROONS

Yield: 20 cookies
Preparation Time: 20 minutes
Cooking Time: 20 minutes
Seasons: All

1¼ cups hazelnuts, plus 20 nuts set aside
⅔ cup date or maple sugar
¼ teaspoon salt
1 teaspoon vanilla extract
4 large egg whites

1. Preheat the oven to 350°. Spread the nuts in one layer on an ungreased baking pan. Bake for 8–10 minutes, until the papery skins become crispy. Watch the nuts carefully, as they will burn easily. Remove them from the oven and let cool.

2. Lower the oven temperature to 300°.

3. Place 1¼ cups of hazelnuts, the date or maple sugar, salt, and vanilla extract into a blender or food processor and blend or pulse until the nuts are finely ground.

4. In a medium bowl, beat the egg whites until they form stiff peaks. Fold the egg whites into the nut mixture and incorporate gently but thoroughly. Grease a cookie sheet. Drop by teaspoonfuls onto the greased cookie sheet to form 1-inch cookies. Place a whole hazelnut in the middle of each cookie, pressing it into the dough slightly. Bake for about 20–24 minutes until slightly golden. Cool for a few minutes on the cookie sheet, then transfer to a plate. Delicious for tea time!

VARIATION:

For thumbprint cookies, gently press your thumb in the center of each cookie. Fill each hollow with ½ teaspoon of your favorite fruit preserves or jam.

CLEANSE NOTE:

This recipe is not appropriate for the cleanse.

POACHED FIGS WITH CINNAMON AND CLOVES

Serves 4
Preparation Time: 10 minutes
Cooking Time: 25 minutes
Seasons: Fall/Winter/Spring

juice of 1 lemon
rind of 1 lemon, cut into strips
2 cups water
½ cup maple syrup
2 cinnamon sticks
6 whole cloves
1 tablespoon vanilla extract
12 dried Black Mission figs, halved

Place all ingredients in a pot and bring to a boil. Cover and reduce the heat to medium-low. Simmer until the figs become soft, about 20 minutes. Strain the mixture through a sieve, discarding the cinnamon, cloves, and lemon rind, but reserving the liquid. Serve the figs warm with the cooked liquid.

CLEANSE NOTE:

This recipe is not appropriate for the cleanse.

CRANBERRY-STUFFED PEARS WITH CRUNCH TOPPING

Serves 2
Preparation Time: 15 minutes
Cooking Time: 25–35 minutes
Seasons: Fall/Winter

1 firm Bosc pear, halved
3–4 tablespoons fresh cranberries

TOPPING

¼ cup roasted almonds, crushed
1 teaspoon cinnamon
½ teaspoon cocoa powder
1 teaspoon vanilla extract
1 tablespoon maple syrup
1 teaspoon extra-virgin olive oil
1 tablespoon freshly squeezed lemon juice

1. Preheat the oven to 350°. Cut a small slice off the rounded side of each pear half, so that it will sit flat in a baking dish. With a melon-baller, scoop out most of the flesh from the bulbous end of the pear, leaving a thin edge all around. Place the pears in a shallow baking dish. Fill the cavities with the whole cranberries, approximately 2 tablespoons per pear half.

2. In a small bowl, mix together all the topping ingredients. Spread the mixture evenly on the tops of the two pear halves. Bake for 25–35 minutes, until the pears and cranberries are soft and the topping becomes solidified. Serve warm or at room temperature.

Cleanse Note:

This recipe is not appropriate for the cleanse.

GLOSSARY OF INGREDIENTS

Arrowroot. A white powder derived from the starchy arrowroot tuber. This starch is great for thickening and binding sauces and soups. Dissolve in a small quantity of cold water before adding it to hot liquids.

Bragg. A salt alternative, Bragg Liquid Aminos is a liquid protein concentrate that's derived from soybeans and contains naturally occurring amino acids. Bragg can be used as a less salty replacement for tamari.

Gomasio. This Japanese condiment is made from toasted sesame seeds ground together with sea salt (1 teaspoon salt, 6 tablespoons sesame seeds). It adds great flavor and texture to dishes. You can readily purchase gomasio in the health food store. To make your own, you will need a suribachi, a ceramic bowl lined with ridges for grinding. Pan roast the seeds and salt for about 5 minutes. Transfer to the suribachi and grind with a wooden pestle until the mixture is 80 percent ground. Or use a spice blender and grind until it forms a coarse powder.

Mirin. A sweet rice wine used for cooking. Read the label to be sure that it is not artificially flavored or sweetened.

Miso. A paste made from fermented soybeans and grains, which is used daily in Japan for its ability to aid digestion. Miso comes in a variety of flavors, from the subtle and sweet white miso to the heartier red miso. Avoid boiling, as intense heat will kill miso's healthy enzymes.

Olive oil. Olive oil is produced in many different countries and varies widely in quality and flavor. When purchasing it, select only cold-pressed extra-virgin olive oil to be assured you're getting the best quality oil.

Rice Wrappers. Also known as rice paper, this product is available from an Asian grocer or many health food stores. It comes dried and is usually found in 4-inch and 8-inch diameters. This thin wrapper becomes flexible when moistened and provides a mild-tasting "shell" that can be filled with a variety of ingredients.

Sake. A clear liquid that is made from rice and water and has about 15 percent alcohol content.

Sea Vegetables. Mostly found in their dehydrated form in health food or Asian stores, these vegetables are harvested from different oceans of the world. People who live in coastal regions have eaten sea vegetables for thousands of years, benefiting from their high content of vitamins and minerals. There are myriad types of sea vegetables, some of which are defined here, all of which fall into one of four categories: Brown Algae, Green Algae, Red Algae, or Blue-Green Algae. It is generally best to rinse, if not soak, the sea vegetables prior to using them. But don't discard the soaking water—use it for your plants. People aren't the only ones who can benefit from the rich vitamins and minerals.

> **Arame.** This mild-tasting sea vegetable is a member of the Brown Algae family. Arame is high in calcium and potassium. Because the plant's large fronds are cooked well and shredded thinly before dehydration, arame requires only a quick soaking in water before using in recipes.

> **Dulse.** This sea vegetable has a beautiful deep red color, strong flavor, and delicate leaves. This Red Algae is high in potassium and can be purchased in strips or in "sprinkles," making it a versatile garnish for soups and vegetables. When using the leaves in strips, only a quick rinse is required before use.

> **Hiziki.** A hearty-flavored member of the Brown Algae family and high in calcium, hiziki requires 15–20 minutes of soaking prior to

use. It stands up well to cooking and baking, and is delicious with hearty vegetables such as squash and root vegetables.

Kelp. A large family of sea vegetables that includes wakame, arame, and kombu, this Brown Algae has large, flat, smooth fronds and is found both on the Pacific and Atlantic coasts of North America. Because its leaves double in size when reconstituted, only small pieces are needed to enhance the flavor of the ingredients it's cooked with. It is rich in iodine, calcium, iron, and potassium.

Nori. Also known as Sea Laver, nori is a member of the Red Algae family. A source of protein, calcium, and iron, it is usually sold in the form of paperlike sheets and is most commonly used for sushi rolls. Nori can easily be cut up into pieces or strips to be used as a garnish for soups and vegetable dishes.

Wakame. This member of the Brown Algae family is rich in minerals and can be purchased in strips or in pre-crumbled bits. It can be eaten raw after a quick soak in water. Wakame is mostly known for its use in miso soups, but also makes a great garnish for fish and vegetables. Or eat the crumbled bits right out of the bag for a delicious, crunchy, and salty snack.

Tamari. This versatile salty condiment is a staple for Asian cooking. The traditional method of making tamari is to extract and age the soybean liquid that rises to the top of miso vats. When purchasing tamari, look for the wheat-free variety.

Wasabi. Japanese in origin, this spicy and pungent root (similar to horseradish root) is in the mustard family. It is usually grated and prepared into a paste that is used as a key ingredient in sauces and dressings, and as a condiment for sushi.

SELECTED BIBLIOGRAPHY

Barks, Coleman, John Moyne, A. J. Arberry, and Reynold Nicholson, trans. *The Essential Rumi*. San Francisco: HarperCollins, 1995.

Berg, Stephen, trans. *Crow with No Mouth: Ikkyū, 15th Century Zen Master, Versions by Stephen Berg*. Port Townsend, WA: Copper Canyon Press, 1989.

Campbell, Joseph, and Bill Moyers. *The Power of Myth*. Edited by Betty Sue Flowers. New York: Doubleday, 1988.

Cleary, Thomas, trans. *The Taoist Classics, Volume 3*. Boston: Shambhala, 2000.

Haas, Elson M., M.D. *Staying Healthy with the Seasons*. Berkeley: Celestial Arts, 1981.

Heschel, Abraham Joshua. *God in Search of Man: A Philosophy of Judaism*. New York: The Noonday Press, 1955.

Lao Tzu. *Tao Te Ching*. Translated by Stephen Mitchell. New York: Harper and Row, 1988.

Metzger, Deena. *Writing for Your Life: A Guide and Companion to the Inner Worlds*. San Francisco: HarperCollins, 1992.

Nelson, Richard K., Kathleen H. Mautner, and G. Ray Bane. *Tracks in the Wildland: A Portrayal of Koyukon and Nunamiut Subsistence*. Fairbanks: Anthropology and Historic Preservation, Cooperative Park Studies Unit, University of Alaska, 1982.

Nestle, Marion. *Food Politics: How the Food Industry Influences Nutrition and Health*. Berkeley: University of California Press, 2002.

Pitchford, Paul. *Healing with Whole Foods: Oriental Traditions and Modern Nutrition*. Berkeley: North Atlantic Books, 1993.

Ray, Paul H., Ph.D., and Sherry Ruth Anderson, Ph.D. *The Cultural Creatives: How 50 Million People Are Changing the World*. New York: Harmony Books, 2000.

Redmond, Layne. *When the Drummers Were Women: A Spiritual History of Rhythm*. New York: Three Rivers Press, 1997.

Rilke, Rainer Maria. *Letters to a Young Poet*. Translated by M. D. Herter Norton. New York: W. W. Norton and Company, 1954.

Schlosser, Eric. *Fast Food Nation: The Dark Side of the All-American Meal*. Boston: Houghton Mifflin Company, 2001.

Snyder, Gary. *The Practice of the Wild*. San Francisco: North Point Press, 1990.

Spangler, David. *The Call*. New York: Riverhead Books, 1996.

Swami Chidvilasananda. *The Yoga of Discipline*. South Fallsburg, NY: SYDA Foundation, 1996.

Veith, Ilza, trans. *The Yellow Emperor's Classic of Internal Medicine*. Berkeley: University of California Press, 1972.

Willet, Walter, with P. J. Skerrett. *Eat, Drink, and Be Healthy: The Harvard Medical School Guide to Healthy Eating*. New York: Simon & Schuster, 2001.